AIDS-ASSOCIATED SYNDROMES

ADVANCES IN EXPERIMENTAL MEDICINE AND BIOLOGY

Recent Volumes in this Series

Volume 182
GENE EXPRESSION IN MUSCLE
Edited by Richard C. Strohman and Stewart Wolf

Volume 183
DRUGS AFFECTING LIPID METABOLISM VIII
Edited by David Kritchevsky, William L. Holmes, and Rodolfo Paoletti

Volume 184
MECHANISMS OF CELL-MEDIATED CYTOTOXICITY II
Edited by Pierre Henkart and Eric Martz

Volume 185
IMMUNOBIOLOGY OF PROTEINS AND PEPTIDES III: VIRAL AND BACTERIAL ANTIGENS
Edited by M. Zouhair Atassi and Howard L. Bachrach

Volume 186
MICROENVIRONMENTS IN THE LYMPHOID SYSTEM
Edited by G. G. B. Klaus

Volume 187
AIDS-ASSOCIATED SYNDROMES
Edited by Sudhir Gupta

Volume 188
SOMATOSTATIN
Edited by Yogesh C. Patel and Gloria S. Tannenbaum

A Continuation Order Plan is available for this series. A continuation order will bring delivery of each new volume immediately upon publication. Volumes are billed only upon actual shipment. For further information please contact the publisher.

AIDS-ASSOCIATED SYNDROMES

Edited by
Sudhir Gupta
California College of Medicine
University of California
Irvine, California

PLENUM PRESS • NEW YORK AND LONDON

Library of Congress Cataloging in Publication Data

International Conference on AIDS-Associated Syndromes (1984: Irvine, Calif.)
AIDS-associated syndromes.

(Advances in experimental medicine and biology; v. 187)
"Proceedings of the International Conference on AIDS-Associated Syndromes, held December 8-9, 1984, in Irvine, California"—T.p. verso.
Includes bibliographies and index.
1. Acquired immune deficiency syndrome—Congresses. I. Gupta, Sudhir. II. Title. III. Series. [DNLM: 1. Acquired Immunodeficiency Syndrome—congresses. W1 AD559 v.187/WD 308 I604a 1984]
RC607.A26I58 1984 616.9′792 85-9468
ISBN-13: 978-1-4615-9432-1 e-ISBN-13: 978-1-4615-9430-7
DOI: 10.1007/978-1-4615-9430-7

Proceedings of the International Conference on AIDS-Associated Syndromes, held December 8-9, 1984, in Irvine, California

Softcover reprint of the hardcover 1st edition 1985
A Division of Plenum Publishing Corporation
233 Spring Street, New York, N.Y. 10013

PREFACE

This is the proceedings of the International Conference on AIDS-Associated Syndromes held at Irvine on December 7-8, 1984. The purpose of this conference was to bring together investigators who are actively engaged in AIDS research to present their most recent data with regard to etiological agent(s) of AIDS, immunological characteristics of some of the patients in early stages of AIDS and various therapeutical modalities that are available for the treatment of AIDS, early AIDS (persistent generalized lymphadnopathy) or for those who demonstrate asymptomatic acquired immunodeficiency.

In the area of etiological agents, the discussions are presented dealing with the questions of whether HTLV III/LAV alone or with other co-factor(s) like EBV or CMV are responsible for AIDS. What is the relationship of these viruses to Kaposi's sarcoma, since Kaposi's sarcoma in AIDS cannot be simply explained on the basis of the underlying immune deficiency? Data are presented for HTLV III/LAV interactions with the T4 molecule on the surface of helper T cells. A paper is presented with epidemiological evidence for AIDS being an African disease which perhaps was brought to the United States and then to Haiti.

In the area of persistent generalized lymphadenopathy syndrome, longitudinal immunological studies are presented to determine whether this clinical spectrum is a precursor of full-blown AIDS as defined by surveillance criteria, or a distinct clinical entity. If so, what are the clinical, cellular, and/or serological markers that determine the outcome of this disorder?

The third and last area focuses on various modes of treatments of AIDS, persistent generalized lymphadenopathy syndrome and asymptomatic subjects who show in vitro immune deficiency. Some of these agents are cytotoxic and work directly on Kaposi's sarcoma, while others are immunomodulators. A new syndrome of oral viral leukoplakia associated with AIDS is introduced.

Sudhir Gupta

CONTENTS

AIDS - AN AFRICAN DISEASE?

Kevin M. De Cock

USC Liver Unit
Rancho Los Amigos Hospital
Downey, California

Introduction:

Compelling evidence exists incriminating the lymphotropic retroviruses LAV[1] (lymphadenopathy associated virus) and HTLV-III[2] (human T lymphotropic virus-III) as the causative agents of the acquired immunodeficiency syndrome (AIDS). Understandably, research has concentrated on elucidating the cause of AIDS, studying its immunology and clinical features, and establishing its epidemiology. There are a number of broad questions that still deserve consideration: (1) Is this a new disease? (2) Why has it appeared now? (3) Why is it specifically associated with Kaposi's sarcoma (KS)? (4) What is the association with Haiti? (5) Why does it affect homosexuals, drug users and haemophiliacs? (6) What is the significance of the increasing number of black African cases?

This paper discusses the hypothesis that AIDS is a Central African disease that recently disseminated into external populations.[3] Attention is drawn to some similarities between the complications of AIDS and the pattern of disease in Sub-Saharan Africa, and a literature review of African AIDS and the role of retroviruses is presented.

Is AIDS a New Disease?

The current epidemic of Kaposi's sarcoma and opportunistic infections in the United States and Western Europe is clearly a new phenomenon. Many initially believed that some new organism or mutant was responsible. We have, however, no examples of genuinely new infectious organisms, and when microbial agents undergo genetic change to enhance their survival, the resulting illnesses are rarely significantly different. In general, when "new" infections are recognized (Table 1), it is clear in retrospect how they existed undetected.

Table 1. Some Recently Recognized Infectious Diseases

- Legionnaire's disease
- Toxic shock syndrome
- Delta hepatitis
- Epidemic, water-borne, non-A, non-B hepatitis
- *Schistosoma mekongi* infection

An illness as impressive as AIDS would not pass unnoticed in the West, and it is unlikely that it could have been harboured in Western homosexual communities for any length of time. A change in its epidemiology rather than in its underlying nature is likely to have brought the AIDS agent to attention.

Certain recently described African viral haemorrhagic fevers demonstrate how impressive infections may remain undetected until a change in the pattern of disease brings them to medical attention. Lassa fever[4] was recognized because American missionary workers contracted the disease, while Marburg virus[5] came to light when transmission of infection occurred from monkeys to laboratory staff in Europe. Subsequent documented outbreaks[6,7] affected white expatriates and hospital staff (Table 2). Ebola haemorrhagic fever was detected in Southern Sudan[8] and Northern Zaire[9] when it occurred in epidemic form (Table 3). Seroepidemiological investigations have shown that these infections must occur sporadically in indigenous rural populations, but diagnosis depends on access to sophisticated medical care.

In rural Africa diagnosis is frequently inexact. Infectious diseases remain the major cause of death, and sporadic immunodeficiency would go unrecognized. If AIDS has been recognized in African cities recently, it is because the condition was specifically looked for, the number of cases was striking, and more extensive investigative facilities are available in urban centres for the diagnosis of opportunistic infections. Few viral illnesses cause disease in every infected individual, and extensive seroepidemiological investigations are indicated to assess patterns of infection with LAV/HTLV III. A rural African origin for AIDS deserves consideration.

Table 2. Marburg Virus Disease

Year	Place	Cases	Deaths	(%)
1977	West Germany Yugoslavia	31	7	(22.6)
1975	South Africa	3	1	(33.3)
1980	Kenya	3	1	(33.3)

Table 3. Ebola Haemorrhagic Fever

Year	Place	Cases	Deaths	(%)
1976	Southern Sudan	284	151	(53)
1976	Northern Zaire	318	280	(88)

Kaposi's Sarcoma and Other Complications of AIDS

Experience with immunosuppressed patients such as organ transplant recipients has yielded a few cases but not an epidemic of KS. The tumour is likely to have a specific cause, rather than simply developing under conditions of impaired tumour surveillance.

Until recently, KS had been a rare tumour in Europe and North America, indolent in nature, most often affecting elderly men of Jewish or Mediterranean origin. It is considerably commoner in Africa, the epicentre being in North-Eastern and Eastern Zaire, where KS accounts for up to 12.8% of all cancers.[10] Table 4 lists various African countries in order of prevalence of KS. The frequency of KS decreases in all directions away from Zaire.

Table 4. Order of Prevalence of KS in Africa

1. Zaire
2. Rwanda/Burundi
3. "French Equatorial Africa"
4. Tanzania
5. Uganda
6. Malawi
7. Zimbabwe
8. Kenya
9. Transvaal (South Africa)
10. Zambia

(from Hutt, 1981)[11]

Surprisingly little attention has been paid to the geographical pathology of KS in the study of AIDS. Other long term complications of tropical infections, such as tropical splenomegaly syndrome or hepatocellular carcinoma, occur elsewhere but KS (possibly causally related to CMV infection) occurs in high incidence only in sub-Saharan Africa. This should be a significant observation.

The clinical patterns of KS are shown in Table 5. Until the recent epidemic the more aggressive varieties of disease were more often seen in African than non-African patients, although the more benign, nodular variety predominated in Africans also.[12] The generalised form of KS has been seen most frequently in children or young people, making up 5 - 10% of cases.

Table 5. Clinical Patterns of Kaposi's Sarcoma

1. Nodular	
2. Aggressive	
	Exophytic (ulcerative)
	Infiltrative
3. Generalized	
	Lymphadenopathic
	Gastrointestinal
	Systemic

(from Templeton, 1981[12])

Immunological function in African KS has received limited attention (Table 6).[13-15] It would seem from the few studies available that cellular immunity is deficient in the aggressive forms of KS. A recent Zambian article[16] documented a local increase in the number of cases with aggressive KS, as well as reversal of T helper to T suppressor cell ratios. The relevance of these findings to AIDS is unclear.

Table 6. Immunological Function in African Kaposi's Sarcoma

Master et al, 1970[13]	Normal antibody responses, normal immunoglobulin levels. Impaired delayed hypersensitivity to dinitro- chlorobenzene in aggressive KS.
Taylor, 1973[14]	Impaired PHA-stimulated lymphocyte transformation.
Taylor & Ziegler, 1974[15]	Reduced cutaneous hypersensitivity.
Downing et al, 1984[16]	Reduced T helper/T suppressor cell ratios.

KS is strikingly more common in homosexual than heterosexual patients with AIDS [17], and is no more frequent in African AIDS patients than in heterosexual Western cases. Clearly, AIDS and KS do not result from the same infectious agent, as has been proposed.[18] However, it is possible that the same agent is responsible for endemic KS as for KS in AIDS, but that for some reason this agent is more prevalent or acting differently in homosexual compared with heterosexual AIDS patients. A comparison of patterns of CMV infection in different patient groups with and at risk for AIDS would be worthwhile.

Burkitt's lymphoma (BL) and B cell, non-Hodgkin's lymphoma have both been described with increased frequency in AIDS.[19,20] Although it occurs elsewhere, BL is most common in areas constituting a band across Africa, the "lymphoma belt", 15° North and South of the Equator.[21] This encompasses some of the areas where KS is endemic, although the distribution of Burkitt's tumour, unlike that of KS, is affected by the climatic determinants of malaria.[22] Other forms of lymphoma, particularly non-Hodgkin's lymphoma of the B cell type, also seem particularly common in sub-Saharan Africa. In Kenya, for example, lymphoma is the third most common solid malignancy, after carcinoma of the skin and cervix.[23]

There are a number of tumours common in Africa for which at least some evidence exists favouring a viral aetiology. These include hepatocellular carcinoma, Burkitt's lymphoma, KS, carcinoma of the cervix and carcinoma of the penis. The relevant viruses are HBV, Epstein-Barr virus (EBV), CMV and Herpes simplex. These same viral infections are ubiquitous in the AIDS population, and some analagous tumours have become frequent in male homosexuals suffering from AIDS (Table 7). An understanding of some of these "African" diseases might clarify the pathogenesis of some of the complications of AIDS.

Table 7. Neoplastic Conditions of Increased Incidence in Homosexual Men

Kaposi's sarcoma

B cell, non-Hodgkin's lymphoma

Oropharyngeal, squamous cell carcinoma

Cloacogenic carcinoma

The Association with Haiti

The occurrence of AIDS in Haitians is difficult to explain. AIDS has been seen in Haiti since 1979, and only one case of KS was documented there before that time.[24] The epidemic of AIDS in the United States probably began in 1978,[25] and there is no evidence that the condition occurred in Haiti before the North American outbreak. The ecology of Haiti resembles that of other Caribbean countries, and there is no reason why an endemic viral disease should localise itself to one island. If AIDS were traditionally endemic in Haiti, cases would have been expected in the neighbouring Dominican Republic and elsewhere in the Caribbean. The number of AIDS cases in the United States continues to increase in all patient groups, but the rate of increase is now significantly lower in Haitians than in other groups at high risk.[26] It seems most likely that AIDS was introduced into Haiti from outside, and that sexual activity has since been important in its spread.

An increasing number of well documented cases of AIDS have been reported in black Africans, mainly Zaireans, without obvious risk factors (see below). Three possible cases of AIDS were seen prior to the present epidemic:

1. A Danish surgeon died of *Pneumocystis* pneumonia in Denmark in 1977. She was anergic and also suffered oral candidiasis. She had been working in Zaire, where she became ill in 1976 with chronic diarrhoea, fever, weight loss and generalized lymphadenopathy.[27]

2. A woman from Kinshasa sought medical advice in Belgium in 1977 for her child who was suffering, like two siblings who had previously died, from oral candidiasis. The child showed a depressed cell mediated response. The mother herself became ill, was anergic and died with multiple opportunistic infections early in 1978.[28]

3. A woman from Zaire was seen in Belgium in 1982 with symptoms typical of the prodrome of AIDS. Symptoms dated back to 1979. Her husband had died in Belgium in 1976 from *Salmonella enteritidis* infection and *Candida albicans* pneumonia.[29]

These cases raise the possibility that AIDS may have occurred in Africa before the current Western epidemic.

African AIDS: A Literature Review

In Europe, 21% of patients with AIDS have been Africans,[30] many of whom travelled to Europe specifically to seek medical advice. Prospective studies in Rwanda[31] and Zaire[32] have identified a high incidence of AIDS in the capital cities of these two countries. A recent increase has been noted in Kigali in the number of cases of oesophageal candidiasis,[31] and in Kinshasa in the incidence of central nervous system cryptococcosis.[33] Although the exact significance of these observations is unclear, many of these cases are believed to be associated with AIDS. An increase in the number of cases of aggressive KS in young men was recently reported from Zambia,[34] and immunological abnormalities analogus to those in AIDS were documented.[16] Since KS is endemic in this region, diagnosis of AIDS with KS as the sole manifestation will be difficult to substantiate.

A review of the literature of African AIDS[27-29,31,32,35-41] yielded 85 cases that could be meaningfully analysed. The Zambian cases of KS referred to above,[16,34] the cases described in the report on the epidemiology of AIDS in Europe,[30] and the clusters reported by Piot et al[32] (see below) are not included in this analysis because of lack of data.

Epidemiology: The countries of origin of the 85 cases are shown in table 8. Additional countries from which cases in Europe[30] have originated are Gabon, Congo and Cameroon. The prospective studies from Rwanda[31] and Zaire[32] yielded estimates of annual incidence of 80/100,000 and 17/100,000 respectively. The authors comment that if these estimates are correct, the proportions of the current epidemics in Kinshasa and Kigali exceed those in the major American cities affected.

Table 8. Countries of Origin of African AIDS Cases (December 1984):

Country	Cases	%
Zaire	63	74
Rwanda	17	1.2
Burundi	1	1.2
Chad	1	1.2
Mali	1	1.2
Uganda	1	1.2
Zambia	1	1.2
TOTAL	85	100

Clinical and Demographic Data: Demographic and clinical data are shown in Table 9. Eighty-three of the cases were adults and two were children. The ratio of males to females was 1.2. Fifty-five (64.7%) were diagnosed in Africa and thirty (34.3%) in Europe. Four of the patients were Europeans who had lived in Africa. A case fatality rate of 53.7% was calculated from those cases for which adequate follow-up data were given.

Table 9. Demographic and Clinical Data on African AIDS (December 1984)

Adult	83	
Child	2	Mean Adult Age: 33 years (range 13-56 years)
Male	47	
Female	38	Mean Child Age: 19 months (range 14-24 months)
Black	81	
White	4	

DEATHS: 36/67 (53.7%)

The major manifestation of African AIDS was opportunistic infection (Table 10). KS was less frequent in African patients than in Western homosexual cases, and its prevalence was of the same order as in heterosexual patients with AIDS in the United States.

Table 10. Manifestations of African AIDS (December 1984)

Disease Catagory	Cases	%
Kaposi's sarcoma	2	2.4
Kaposi's sarcoma and Opportunistic infection	11	12.9
Opportunistic infection	72	84.7

The opportunistic and associated infections complicating the African AIDS cases are listed in Table 11 in their order of frequency.

Table 11. Infections in African AIDS (December 1984)

Organisms	Number	% of All Infections
Candida	51	34.9
Herpes	22	15.1
Cryptococcus	18	12.3
Cytomegalovirus	14	9.6
Mycobacteria	10	6.8
Pneumocystis	8	5.5
Salmonella	7	4.8
Toxoplasma	5	3.4
Pseudomonas	3	2.1
Stronglyloides	2	1.4
Entamoeba	1	0.7
Cryptosporidium	1	0.7
Aspergillus	1	0.7
Nocardia	1	0.7
Staphylococcus	1	0.7
Escherichia coli	1	0.7

The low prevalence of Pneumocystis carinii infection may in part reflect the difficulty of making this diagnosis. Open lung or bronchoscopic biopsy is not generally available in African hospitals. A number of patients had undiagnosed, interstitial lung infiltrates, and Pneumocystis infection may have been more frequent than documented. However, in the European experience with AIDS,[42] African cases were also more often complicated by cryptococosis, candidiasis, toxoplasmosis and tuberculosis than by Pneumocystis infection.

AIDS Related Conditions. Many reports mention patients with prodomal symptoms of AIDS. Demographic data were not different from patients with frank AIDS (Table 12).

Table 12. African AIDS Related Conditions (December 1984)

Symptoms: Lymphadenopathy, fever, weight loss, chronic diarrhoea

Male		9	(64.3%)
Female		5	(35.7%)
TOTAL	14	(100%)	

Mean Age 36.7 years (range 24-60)

Risk Factors: None of the 85 patients were known to be intravenous drug users or homosexuals. Blood transfusion was not a risk factor. Scarification and injection with previously used syringes and needles are frequent practices in Africa. No evidence was found that either of these was relevant, although they provide a theoretical mode of transmission, as do insect vectors.

Patients were generally of upper or middle class and lived an urban life-style. The studies from Rwanda[31] and Zaire[32] suggested heterosexual promiscuity was the main risk factor, and strongly supported the concept of heterosexual transmission. In those studies some of the women were prostitutes, while many of the men had frequent sexual contact with different partners, including prostitutes. One woman with generalized lymphadenopathy was the wife of a man with AIDS, while the husbands of two female cases died with AIDS in the six months before the studies.

Piot et al[32] retrospectively identified two clusters of AIDS in heterosexual Zairean partners, all of whom died (Fig 1). These observations, the authors comment, support male to female as well as female to male transmission.

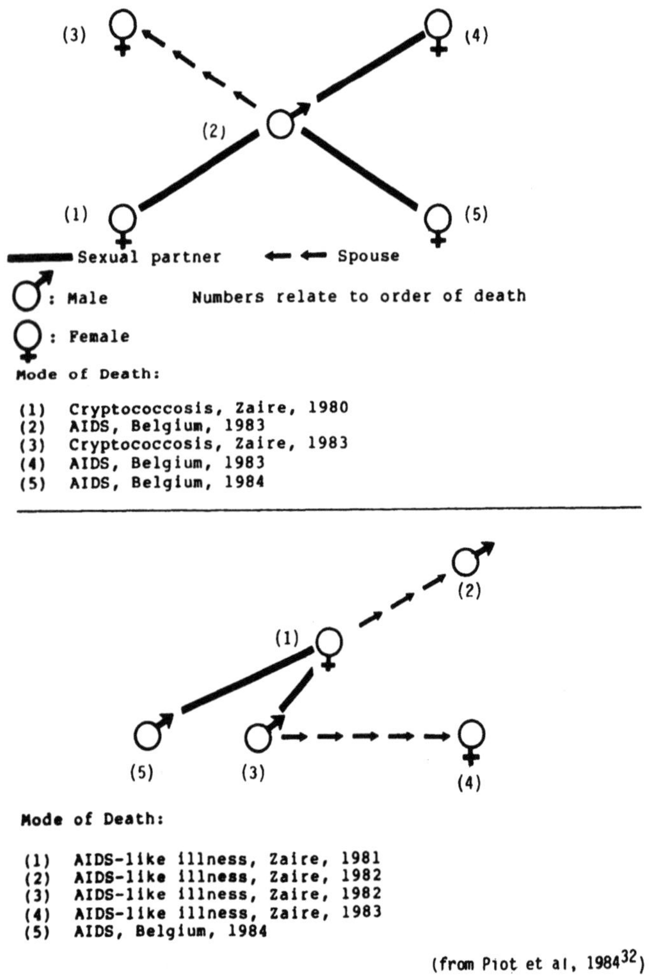

Fig. 1 African Aids Clusters

Lymphotropic Retrovirus Infection in African AIDS

In Africa, infection with human T cell leukaemia- lymphoma virus (HTLV-I) is geographically widespread, although generally of low prevalence.[43-45] Isolated cases of lymphoproliferative disease related to HTLV-I infection have been reported.[45-47] An African origin for the HTLV family has been proposed and discussed elsewhere.[48]

The development of the hypothesis that LAV/HTLV-III is causally linked to AIDS has been reviewed by Broder and Gallo.[49] At the time of writing, the following has been published concerning retrovirus infection in African AIDS:

(1) Belgian workers[50] described virus-like particles on electron microscopy of lymphocytes of African AIDS patients. These particles were claimed to resemble retrovirus particles that had been described in other cases of AIDS.

(2) The lymphotropic retrovirus LAV was isolated from the lymphocytes of a Zairean married couple,[40] of whom the man had AIDS and the woman the prodrome. Specific antibodies were detected in both their sera.

(3) A Zambian nurse who died with AIDS in Britain was subsequently shown to have antibodies to HTLV-III.[41]

(4) None of the 14 patients with KS in Eastern Zaire had antibodies to HTLV-III, while the antibody rate in a control population was 12.4%.[51] This suggests that HTLV-III infection is endemic in Zaire, but that it is not associated with classic KS.

(5) The presence of antibodies to LAV was shown in 35 of 37 (94%) Zairean patients[52] diagnosed as having AIDS in the study from Kinshasa[32] previously referred to. Five of 100 sera collected from a group of Zairean mothers in 1980 were positive, as were 7 of 100 sera from another control group in 1983.

A possible case of AIDS dating back to 1977,[28] a Zairean woman who died in 1978, and who had travelled to Belgium to seek medical care of her child, has retrospectively been shown to have antibodies to LAV.[52] The child is now healthy but one year ago was still weakly sero-positive.

Conclusions:

Despite widespread agreement about the cause of AIDS, broad questions about its origins and sudden appearance remain. Its major modes of transmission, sexual activity or contact with blood, explain the Western risk groups, the same that are commonly affected by hepatitis B infection. In retrospect, undue emphasis may have been placed on the observation that three quarters of Western AIDS patients are homosexuals. Viruses do not infect selectively on the basis of nationality or sexual preference, and Western patterns of LAV/HTLV-III infection may be misleading about the overall epidemiology of the infection, as they are in the case of hepatitis B.

There is an obvious need for further work in different African countries to assess the proportions of the AIDS epidemic there, and to determine the relationship, if any, between certain classical "African" diseases and this "new" syndrome. Only prospective studies will establish the epidemiology of LAV/HTLV-III infection, including its diverse modes of transmission. Without an understanding of such issues, attempts at prevention are unlikely to be successful. That AIDS is an African disease remains the most plausible hypothesis explaining the sudden emergence of this condition.

References:

1. Barre-Sinoussi F, Chermann JC, Rey F, et al. Isolation of a T lymphotropic retrovirus from a patient at risk for acquired immune deficiency syndrome (AIDS). Science 1983, 220:868-870.
2. Gallo RC, Salahuddin SZ, Popoic M, et al. Frequent detection and isolation of cytopathic retroviruses (HTLV-III) from patients with AIDS and at risk for AIDS. Science 1984; 224:500-502.
3. De Cock KM. AIDS: An old disease from Africa? Br Med J 1984, 289:306-308.
4. Frame JD, Baldwin JM, Gocke DJ, Troup JM. Lassa fever, a new virus disease of man from West Africa. I. Clinical description and pathological findings. Am J Trop Med Hyg 1970, 19:670-676.
5. Martini GA, Siegart R, eds. Marburg virus disease. Berlin: Springer Verlag 1971.
6. Gear JSS, Cassel GA, Gear AJ, et al. Outbreak of Marburg virus disease in Johannesburg. Br Med J 1975, 4:489-493.
7. Smith DH, Johnson BK, Isaacson M, et al. Marburg virus disease in Kenya. Lancet 1982, 1:816-820.
8. WHO International Study Team. Ebola haemorrhagic fever in Sudan, 1976. Bull WHO 1978, 56:247-270.
9. International Commission. Ebola haemorrhagic fever in Zaire, 1976. Bull WHO 1978, 56:271-293.
10. Oettle AS. Geographical and racial differences in the frequency of Kaposi's sarcoma as evidence of environmental or genetic causes. Acta Un Int Cancer 1962, 18:330-363.
11. Hutt MSR. The epidemiology of Kaposi's sarcoma. Antibiot Chemother 1981, 29:3-8.
12. Templeton AC. Kaposi's sarcoma. IN: Sommers SC, Rosen PP, eds. Pathology Annual, Appleton-Century-Crofts, New York, 1981, 16, part 2, 315-336.
13. Master SP, Taylor JF, Kyalwazi SK, Ziegler JL. Immunological studies in Kaposi's sarcoma in Uganda. Br Med J 1970, 600-602.
14. Taylor JF. Lymphocyte transformation in Kaposi's sarcoma. Lancet, 1973, 1:883-884.
15. Taylor JF, Ziegler JL. Delayed cutaneous hypersensi- tivity reactions in patients with Kaposi's sarcoma. Br J Cancer 1974, 30:312-318.
16. Downing RG, Eglin RP, Bayley AC. African Kaposi's sarcoma and AIDS. Lancet 1984, 1:478-480.
17. Anonymous. Update. Acquired immunodeficiency syndrome (AIDS) - United States. MMWR 1984, 33:337-339.
18. Weber J. Is AIDS an epidemic form of African Kaposi's sarcoma? Discussion paper. J Roy Soc Med 1984, 77:572-576.
19. Ziegler JL, Drew WL, Miner RC, et al. Outbreak of Burkitt's-like lymphoma in homosexual men. Lancet 1982, 2:631-633.
20. Ziegler JL, Beckstead JA, Volberding PA, et al. Non-Hodgkins' lymphoma in 90 homosexual men. N Engl J Med 1984, 311:565-570.
21. Burkitt DP. Geographical distribution. In: Burkitt DP, Wright DH eds. Burkitt's Lymphoma. Edingburgh: Livingstone, 1970, 186-197.
22. Cook PJ, Burkitt DP. Cancer in Africa. Br Med Bull 1971, 27:14-20.
23. Kungu A, Gatei DG. Kaposi's sarcoma in Kenya. Antibiot Chemother 1981, 29:38-55.
24. Pape JW, Liautaud B, Thomas F, et al. Characteristics of the acquired immunodeficiency syndrome (AIDS) in Haiti. N Engl J Med. 1983, 309:945-950.

25. Centers for Disease Control Task Force on Kaposi's Sarcoma and Opportunistic Infections. Epidemiologic aspects of the current outbreaks of Kaposi's sarcoma and opportunistic infections. N Engl J Med 1982, 306:248-252.
26. Anonymous. Update: Acquired Immunodeficiency Syndrome (AIDS) - United States. MMWR 1974, 33:661-663.
27. Bygbjerg IC. AIDS in a Danish surgeon (Zaire, 1976). Lancet 1983, 1:925.
28. Vandepitte J, Verwilghen R, Zachee P. AIDS and cryptococcosis (Zaire 1977). Lancet 1983, 1:925-926.
29. Clumeck N, Sonnet J, Taelman H, et al. Acquired immunodeficiency syndrome in African patients. N Engl J Med 1984, 310:492-497.
30. Anonymous. The epidemiology of AIDS in Europe. Eur J Cancer Clin Oncol 1984, 20:157-164.
31. Van de Perre P, Rouvroy D, Lepage P, et al. Acquired immunodeficiency syndrome in Rwanda. Lancet 1984, 2:62-65.
32. Piot P, Quinn TC, Taelman H, et al. Acquired immuno- deficiency syndrome in a heterosexual population in Zaire. Lancet 1984, 2:65-69.
33. Lamey B, Melameka N. Aspects cliniques et epidemiolo- giques de la cryptococcose a Kinshasa: a propos de 15 cas personnels. Med Trop 1982, 42:507-511.
34. Bayley AC. Aggressive Kaposi's sarcoma in Zambia, 1983. Lancet 1984, 1:1318-1320.
35. Clumeck N, Mascart-Lemone F, De Maubeuge J, Brenez D, Marcelis L. Acquired immune deficiency syndrome in black Africans. Lancet 1983, 1:642.
36. Offenstadt G, Pinta P, Hericord P, et al. Multiple opportunistic infection due to AIDS in a previously healthy black woman from Zaire. N Engl J Med 1983, 308:775.
37. Brunet JB, Bouvet E, Leibowitch J, et al. Acquired immunodeficiency syndrome in France. Lancet 1983, 1:700-701.
38. Vittecoq D, Modai J. AIDS in a Black Malian. Lancet 1983, 2:1023-
39. Edwards D, Harper PG, Pain AK, et al. Kaposi's sarcoma associated with AIDS in a woman from Uganda. Lancet 1984, 1:631-632.
40. Ellrodt A, Barre-Sinoussi F, Le Bras PL, et al. Isolation of human T lymphotropic retrovirus (LAV) from Zairean married couple, one with AIDS, one with prodromes. Lancet 1984, 1:1383-1385.
41. Raine AEG, Ilgren EB, Kurtz JB, Ledingham JGG, Waddell JA. HTLV-III infection and AIDS in a Zambian nurse resident in Britain. Lancet 1984, 2:985.
42. Anonymous. Clinical features of AIDS in Europe. Eur J Cancer Clin Oncol 1984, 20:165-167.
43. Saxinger W, Blattner WA, Levine PH, et al. Human T cell leukaemia virus (HTLV-I) antibodies in Africa. Science 1984, 225:1473-1476.
44. Biggar RJ, Saxinger C, Gardiner C, et al. Type-I HTLV antibody in urban and rural Ghana, West Africa. Int J Cancer 1984, 34:215-219.
45. Fleming AF, Yamamoto N, Bhusnurmath SR, et al. Antibodies to ATLV (HTLV) in Nigerian blood donors and patients wth chronic lymphatic leukaemia or lymphoma. Lancet 1983, 2:334-335.
46. Williams CKO, Alabi GO, Junaid TA, et al. Human T cell leukaemia virus associated lymphoproliferative disease: report of two cases in Nigeria. Br Med J 1984, 288:1495-1496.
47. Stewart JSW, Matutes E, Lampert IA, Goolden AWS, Catovsky D. HTLV-I positive T cell lymphoma/leukaemia in an African resident in UK. Lancet 1984, 2:984-985.
48. Gallo RC, Sliski A, Wong-Staal F. Origin of human T-cell leukaemia-lymphoma virus. Lancet 1983, 2:962-963.
49. Broder S, Gallo RC. A pathogenic retrovirus (HTLV-III) linked to AIDS. N Engl J Med 1984, 311:1292-1297.

50. Feremans W, Menu R, Dustin P, Clumeck N, Marcelis L, Hupin J. Virus-like particles in lymphocytes of seven cases of AIDS in Black Africans. Lancet 1984, 2:52-53.
51. Biggar RJ, Melbye M, Kestems L, et al. Kaposi's sarcoma in Zaire is not associated with HTLV-III infection. N Engl J Med 1984, 311:1051-1052.
52. Brun-Vezinet F, Rouzioux C, Montagnier L, et al. Prevalence of antibodies to lymphadenopathy-associated retrovirus in African patients with AIDS. Science 1984, 226:453-456.

ETIOLOGY OF AIDS: BIOLOGICAL AND BIOCHEMICAL CHARACTERISTICS OF HTLV-III

Phillip D. Markham, George M. Shaw, S. Zaki Salahuddin,
Beatrice Hahn, M.G. Sarngadharan, and Robert C. Gallo

Laboratory of Tumor Cell Biology
National Cancer Institute
National Institutes of Health
Bethesda, MD 20205

INTRODUCTION

The human T-cell leukemia (lymphotropic) viruses comprise a group of retroviruses which share several structural, biochemical, and biological properties, and have been collectively named HTLV in accordance with guidelines established by a group of scientists at an international conference on human retroviruses (19,79). The properties shared by all known members of the HTLV group include; 1) tropism for T-lymphocytes, 2) a high molecular weight, Mg+-preferring reverse transcriptase, 3) similar size, number and genomic organization of major core proteins, 4) cytopathic effect on infected cells, 5) prevalence of 3' terminal gene, Lor, and double splicing mechanisms coding for a transactivating protein, 6) distant antigenic and nucleic acid relatedness, and 7) a likely African origin.

Three major subgroups of HTLV have now been identified. The first and most thoroughly studied, named HTLV-I, has been etiologically linked to adult T-cell leukemia (ATL, reviewed in refs. 17, 19). Over 100 isolates have been obtained and, although almost all are identical, some variants, e.g., HTLV-Ib (24), have also been found. A second member of the HTLV group, HTLV-II, which has been only rarely observed, was originally isolated from a cell line established from a patient, MO, with a variant of hairy cell leukemia (33). The third and most recently recognized member of this group of human retroviruses, HTLV-III, is the etiological agent for the Acquired Immunodeficiency Syndrome (AIDS), and its related diseases (18,54).

The HTLV group of retroviruses, therefore, affords the reagents, i.e., etiologic agents, to study and hopefully to eventually understand the mechanism responsible for two human diseases, i.e., ATL and AIDS or its associated syndromes. Details of the characteristics of HTLV-I and HTLV-II have been reviewed elsewhere (17,19) and will be mentioned here only for the purpose of comparison when needed. This presentation presents evidence linking HTLV-III to AIDS, and describes its biological and biochemical properties, including similarities and differences with other members of the HTLV group and other retroviruses.

ISOLATION OF HTLV-III

Soon after the recognition of AIDS and its related syndromes, e.g., AIDS-related complex (ARC) and persistent generalized lymphadenopathy (PGL), as distinct disease entities, it became apparent that they were caused by an infectious agent likely transmitted by repeated close physical contact or by blood or blood products (5,7,15). Several factors also suggested that this agent could be a virus, and possibly a retrovirus similar to HTLV-I and HTLV-II. In addition to similarities in the mode of transmission, the agent responsible for AIDS was filterable, i.e., filtered blood products such as Factor VIII received by hemophiliacs retained the infectious agent, it also had a unique host cell range, i.e., the preferential infection of T4 lymphocytes, and, like HTLV-I, the agent responsible for AIDS also appeared to have an African connection.

Experiments to isolate virus from AIDS and ARC patients and from other donors at risk for these diseases were initiated in 1982 using procedures patterned after those used for the isolation of other members of the HTLV family. Mitogen stimulated human mononuclear cells were grown in the presence of T-cell growth factor (TCGF), also called interleukin-2 (Il-2), and virus was detected by monitoring supernatant fluids for viral reverse transcriptase activity (64), by transmission to fresh normal human adult peripheral blood, bone marrow, or umbilical cord blood T-lymphocytes (18), or to established T-cell lines (53,54). The expression and release of virus was also monitored by electron microscopic observation of fixed, sectioned cells, and by immunofluorescence or radioimmunoprecipitation procedures using serum from sero-positive donors and eventually with specific antisera to viral proteins. As large quantities of virus became available resulting from its transmission to and production by established cell lines (53,54), many HTLV-III-specific immunological and nucleic acid reagents were prepared.

The results of establishing primary cells from patients or donors in cell culture are illustrated in Figure 1. Using cells from an ARC patient, virus is usually detected in supernatant fluids within 2 to 3 weeks after introduction into tissue culture. Release of virus usually declines rapidly coinciding with a loss of viable cells, especially those with the helper/inducer (OKT4/Leu3a+) phenotype. Often a second peak of virus production is observed occurring several weeks after the initial detection of virus. The reason for this second peak is not known, but from an evaluation of the total cell count and the number of OKT4/Leu3a+ cells it appears that a minor population of cells susceptible to HTLV-III infection survive the initial release of virus and are either subsequently infected, or activated, and release virus.

The first HTLV-III isolates were obtained in this laboratory in November 1982, and virus has subsequently been isolated from over 100 AIDS or ARC patients and from healthy individuals at risk for AIDS (18,62). A summary of the isolates of HTLV-III obtained in this laboratory along with some patient information concerning their clinical status and the tissue sources of infected cells is summarized in Table 1. The frequency (number of isolates/number of patients or donors tested) of HTLV-III isolation was ∿50% for AIDS patients, ~80% for ARC patients, and 30% for healthy individuals at risk for AIDS. HTLV-III was not found in more than 150 samples from randomly selected healthy heterosexual donors. The incidence of virus isolation is clearly an underestimate of the number of patients who had been exposed to HTLV-III, since the majority (>90%) of AIDS and ARC patients were seropositive for antibody to HTLV-III proteins (discussed below).

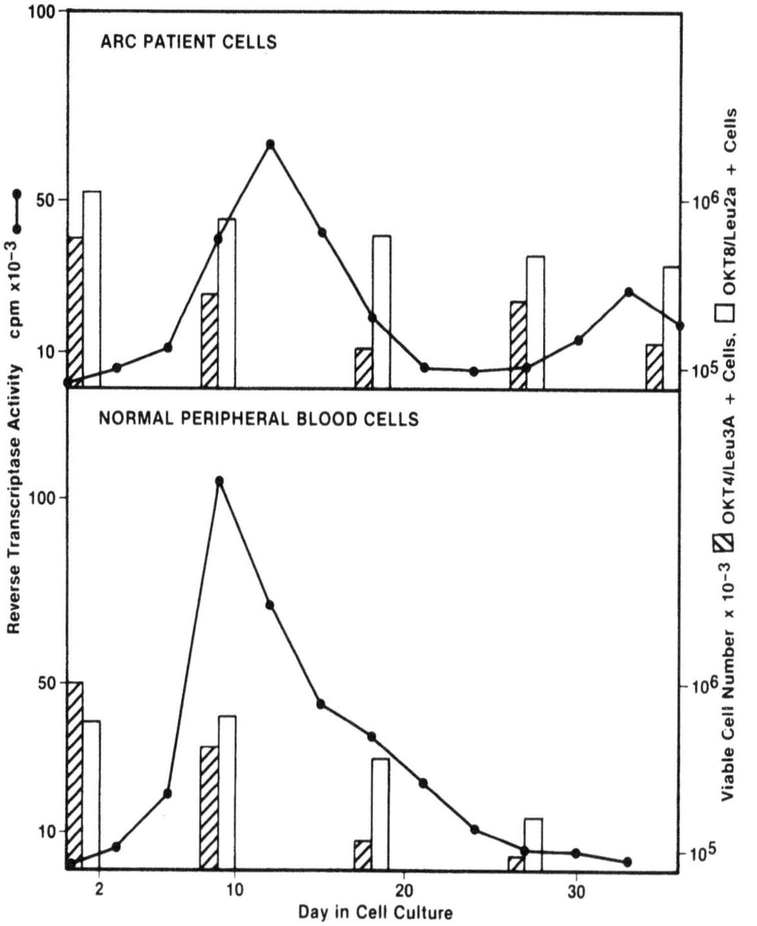

Figure 1. HTLV-III produced by primary cells established in cell culture from an ARC patient (top) and by HTLV-III-infected normal peripheral blood cells (bottom). Top panel. Mononuclear cells were prepared from an ARC patients peripheral blood, treated with PHA-p for 48 hrs, and grown in suspension culture with TCGF. Virus release was monitored by reverse transcriptase activity in supernatant fluids and cell types were determined using cell specific monoclonal antibody. Bottom panel. Fresh mononuclear cells from normal donor were infected by cell-free HTLV-III and monitored as described above.

The morphological appearance of virus (HTLV-III) produced by AIDS/ARC patients and donors at risk for AIDS is shown in Figure 2. HTLV-III is morphologically distinct from HTLV-I or -II, which can also be distinguished from type C retroviruses. Morphologically, HTLV-III resembles members of the Lentivirus family, one characteristic being the formation of bar-shaped nucleoids during maturation (20). Others had suggested resemblances between these viruses and both equine infectious anemia virus (a Lentivirus) and Type D viruses (3,48), however, there is a clear distinction between HTLV-III and type D retrovirus (20). Other similarities between HTLV-III and Lentiviruses include: 1) a cytopathic effect on in vitro infected cells and 2) their ability to produce persistent debilitating diseases in vivo (20).

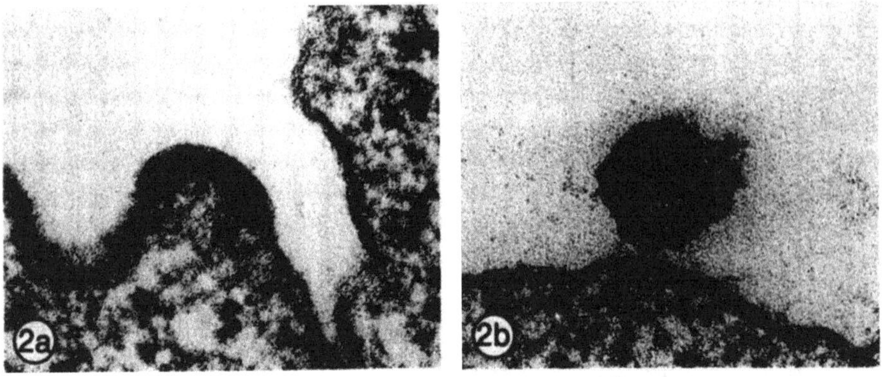

Figure 2. Transmission electron micrograph of HTLV-III-infected human leukocytes A) budding and B) mature virion (150,000X).

TISSUE SOURCES OF INFECTIOUS VIRUS

As shown in Table 1, the majority of HTLV-III isolations to date have been from peripheral blood leukocytes, however, in a smaller number of samples, infectious virus was also isolated from leukocytes obtained from bone marrow and lymph node tissues and, consistent with their probable involvement in AIDS-related encephalopathy and other neurological disorders, from brain tissues (73 and our personal observation). Consistent with its sexual transmission, leukocytes found in the semen of 2 AIDS patients (82) and a healthy homosexual male (30), also produced virus when grown in cell culture. Relevant to the transmission of virus from blood products, HTLV-III was also isolated from cell-free plasma (our personal observation). HTLV-III was also isolated from lymphocytes found in saliva from healthy homosexual men who were at high risk for AIDS, and from ARC patients (21). This suggests that sexual contact or transmission by blood or blood products need not be the only route of transmission to be considered. Even though the spread of virus or disease by casual contact is considered a rare event (29), the presence of virus infected cells in the saliva of these patients and donors suggests that heavy salivary exchange should be considered as a possible risk factor.

The isolation of virus from cultured cells was substantially facilitated by inclusion of hydrocortisone in culture media. For example, in ~50% of samples from virus positive AIDS or ARC patients, the amount of virus released was substantially increased when 5 μg/ml hydrocortisone was used. More importantly, in ~15% of AIDS specimens, the inclusion of hydrocortisone or some other hormone allowed detection of virus that would otherwise have gone undetected (42).

The detection and isolation of a human T-lymphotropic retrovirus from AIDS and ARC patients has also been accomplished independently by others. In addition to the virus, termed lymphoadenopathy associated virus or LAV, detected in leukocytes from an ARC patient by Barré-Sinnousi et al. (3), this same group also reported the isolation of similar viruses which they named immunodeficiency associated virus IDAV-1 and 2 (48). Others have also recently described isolation of these human T-lymphotropic viruses (16,41). Direct genomic comparison between these viruses demonstrates that they are very similar (55,63,78).

TABLE 1

SUMMARY OF DONOR AND TISSUE SOURCE OF HTLV-III ISOLATES

Tissue[2]	Donor/Patient[1] Healthy at Risk	ARC	AIDS
Peripheral blood	16/50	31/38	43/88
Bone Marrow	NT[3]	1/6	NT
Lymph Node	NT	4/4	NT
Brain Biopsy	NT	NT	2/3
Plasma	NT	3/6	NT
Saliva[4]	4/6	4/10	0/4
Semen[5]	1/1	NT	2/2

[1] Healthy; clinically normal individuals from at-risk groups; ARC, AIDS-Related Complex; AIDS, Acquired Immunodeficiency Syndrome. Numbers indicate number of virus isolates per number of donors/patients tested.

[2] With all tissues except plasma, mononuclear cells were prepared and established in cell culture. Cell-free plasma from patients previously identified as virus carriers was used to infect normal human lymphocytes *in vitro*.

[3] NT, Not Tested.

[4] Studies performed in collaboration with Dr. J. Groopman, New England Deaconess Hospital, Boston, MA (21).

[5] Studies performed by Dr. Zagury *et al.*, University of Paris(82), and Drs. D. Ho, M. Hirsch *et al.*, Massachusetts General Hospital, Boston, MA (30).

TRANSMISSION OF HTLV-III BY HETEROSEXUAL CONTACT

Earlier epidemiological observations had suggested that AIDS could be contracted by female sexual partners of male members of high-risk groups. This was noted in a study of AIDS and ARC cases in the U.S. (22,26) and in studies in Africa which demonstrated the almost equal occurrence of these syndromes in men and women (8,51,77). Seroepidemiological tests of donor sera further demonstrated the elevated (36%) incidence of antibodies to HTLV-III in female contacts of AIDS and ARC patients (our personal observations with M. Robert-Guroff), and similar studies revealed a very high incidence (~60%) of HTLV-III serum antibodies in a prostitute population in parts of Africa (our personal observation with C. Saxinger). This male-to-female transmission of virus and consequently disease was directly shown in a case study of seven families where the husband had either AIDS or ARC (56). Five spouses with no other risk factor had evidence of HTLV-III infection documented by seropositivity and/or isolation of virus. Three of these 5 spouces had also developed ARC. Of 11 children belonging to these families only one, a 14 month old child, was seropositive for HTLV-III. The antibody in this one infant was likely a result of congenital infection.

Female-to-male transmission of virus was also suggested in a carefully controlled study involving U.S. military personnel presenting with AIDS or ARC. Seven out of 19 men in this study gave no history linking them to a recognized AIDS risk group. All seven were seropositive for antibody to HTLV-III and infectious virus was isolated from their peripheral blood lymphocytes. The only common factor among these 7 patients was the frequent employment of prostitutes, or other frequent heterosexual contacts (more than 6 encounters with prostitutes per year for 2 consecutive years, or more than 10 different heterosexual partners per year for 2 years). These contacts occurred in various parts of the world, with New York and Germany being frequently mentioned (our personal observation with R. Redfield). These studies suggest that, in addition to concern for the rise of HTLV-III infection and the consequential disease in various parts of the world occurring in AIDS risk groups (discussed below), at least certain heterosexually promiscuous groups should also be followed.

SEROEPIDEMIOLOGY

The etiological association between HTLV-III and AIDS was conclusively established by seroepidemiological evidence. The techniques used to screen serum from a large number of patients and donors for antibodies to HTLV-III included: (a) indirect live cell membrane immunofluorescence (11,12), (b) enzyme-linked immunosorbence assay (ELISA) (65,66,69), (c) Western blot analysis usng patient sera and purified virus (59,65,69), and (d) competition radioimmunoprecipitation using purified HTLV-III structural proteins (32, our personal observation).

In early studies, Essex and co-workers, using a live-cell immunofluorescence assay, found that up to 50% of AIDS patients had serum antibodies that reacted with antigens present on HTLV-I-infected cells (11,12). This was in contrast to less than 1% of healthy homosexuals and immunosuppressed controls. Further investigation indicated that the antigen recognized by these AIDS sera was an epitope of the HTLV-I envelope protein (39). Using solid-phase immunoassays, Robert-Guroff and coworkers found that sera from AIDS and ARC patients possessed antibodies to disrupted HTLV-I (57,58). The conclusion from these two independent observations was that a retrovirus at least distantly related to HTLV-I had widely infected the AIDS population.

Once isolates of the virus became available in large quantities (54), and immunological and other specific probes were prepared, definitive seroepidemiological studies were conducted that confirmed and extended the earlier observations. Sera from AIDS and ARC patients, donors at risk for AIDS, and multiple normal controls were initially screened by ELISA using disrupted purified HTLV-III. ELISA positive sera and those that were questionable or were otherwise considered to be of particular importance were further tested by the more sensitive Western blot procedure. Sera were considered to contain antibody to HTLV-III proteins if they were positive in the Western blot assay even if the results were initially equivocal by ELISA. As viral reagents, such as purified viral proteins and specific antisera, became available quantitative experiments using competition radioimmunoassay were also performed.

The results obtained with a representative number of several thousand sera tested are summarized in Table 2. As indicated, greater than >90% of all AIDS and ARC patients were found seropositive for antibodies to HTLV-III. In contrast, control sera including those from randomly collected healthy donors and people with non-AIDS related illnesses were negative. Others with antibodies to HTLV-III included individuals at risk for acquiring AIDS. For example, promiscuous homosexual men, intravenous drug abusers and recent Haitian immigrants to the U.S. were positive at an incidence much higher than the normal population. Among individuals with no traditional risk factors for AIDS were a selected population of heterosexual promiscuous men (discussed previously), and recipients of multiple transfusions of blood products (31). In fact, a careful screening of blood donors and recipients gave a very conclusive cause-and-effect pattern. For example, all 19 individuals (who were previously healthy, and did not belong to another risk group) who developed AIDS as a result of receiving a blood transfusion from an individual belonging to a defined AIDS risk group were found to have antibodies to HTLV-III. Furthermore, 31 of 35 high-risk donors (who belonged to a AIDS risk group and/or subsequently developed AIDS) who contributed blood to patients were seropositive. Twenty-eight recipients of blood from these donors subsequently developed AIDS.

TABLE 2. Antibodies to HTLV III in sera of patients with AIDS and AIDS related complex

Patients/Donors	Number Positive/Number Tested (%)
Patients with AIDS	288/297 (97)
Patients with ARC	327/360 (91)
Asymptomatic Homosexual Men	96/235 (41)
Transfusion AIDS	19/19 (100)
High-Risk Transfusion Donors	31/35 (87)
Renal Transplant Recipient from High Risk Donor	1/1
Controls	
Normal Donors	0/515
Miscellaneous Patients[a]	0/364
Miscellaneous Patients[a]	0/364

[a]These include randomly collected samples from: Patients with leukemias and other malignancies from HTLV-I endemic areas, schizophrenics, Hodgkin's patients and siblings, renal transplant recipients and other immunosuppressed cases, black women from Baltimore (1962 collection), healthy Japanese from HTLV-I Endemic regions, healthy surinamese (methodone-treatment group) heavily transfused patients and those with: hepatitis B virus infection, primary stage syphilis, rheumatoid arthritis, systemic lupus erythematosus, acute mononucleosis, lymphatic leukemias, B- and T-cell lymphomas, alopecia areata, idiopathic splenomegaly.

An example of a confirmatory Western blot test is shown in Figure 3. Representative patterns of antibody reactions with sera from AIDS and ARC patients and healthy homosexuals at risk demonstrated that the viral protein most consistently detected had a molecular weight of ~41,000. This is believed to be a processed product of the HTLV-III envelope. Less frequently, particularly using sera from clinically healthy at-risk patients or patients with early stage disease, the major HTLV-III internal protein, p24, was also detected. Additional reactivities against antigens of 66,000 and 51,000 molecular weights were also seen in some sera. A wide variation of antibody titer was apparent, although antibody to HTLV-III was usually detected in most patients even before clinical symptoms were recognized. Generally, titers of HTLV-III antibodies were significantly lower in advanced AIDS patients than in ARC patients, or healthy normal, at risk donors. These observations are consistent with the eventual death of target cells and general loss of immune function noted *in vivo*.

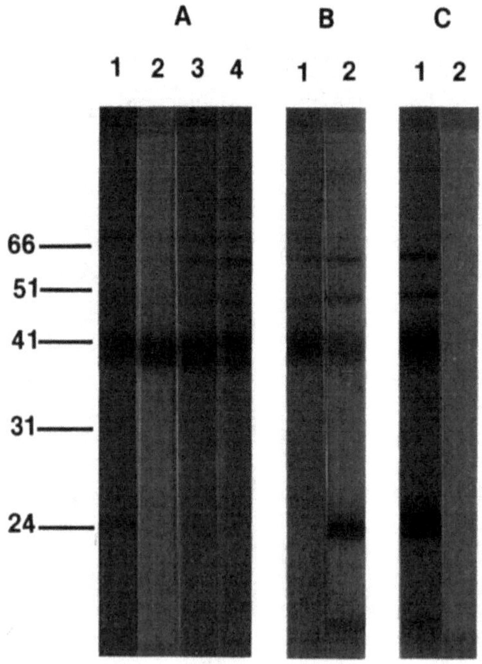

Figure 3. Western Blot analysis of serum from AIDS (A) and ARC (B) patients and from healthy homosexual males at risk for AIDS (C). Proteins from disrupted HTLV-III were electrophoresed on polyacrylamide slab gels, transferred to nitrocellulose paper and incubated with serum from individual donors as previously described.

VIRUS POSITIVE SERONEGATIVE HEALTHY DONORS

Use of serological tests to identify infected invididuals appears to have some limitations. For example, of 101 individuals with AIDS, ARC, or at risk for AIDS from whom infectious virus had been isolated, 4 had no serum antibodies to the virus detectable by any of the assay procedures routinely used (61). Three of these donors were among the approximately 50 clinically healthy, at-risk, group studied. It should be emphasized, however, that these were highly selected individuals, e.g., many were sampled because of specific connections with AIDS or ARC patients, or by referral from clinicians, etc., and may not represent a realistic picture of health, at risk, individuals. Certainly, people falling in this group would represent an infinitesimal portion of all seroneagtive individuals not at risk for AIDS. Since efforts are currently underway to screen blood donors as well as individuals in high risk groups for HTLV-III utilizing assays for antibody, the occurrence of seronegative but virus-positive persons without clinical symptoms does suggest that other assays, possibly based on detection of viral antigens or proviral DNA, may be required in some instances.

WORLDWIDE DISTRIBUTION OF HTLV-III

Despite the need to be aware that some seronegative, virus positive, carriers exists, the high correlation between the presence of serum antibody and disease or risk for developing disease is conclusive. As expected, the correlation between AIDS and ARC ptients, and donors at risk for AIDS and the presence of serum antibody to HTLV-III is the same for specimens collected throughout the world. A greater than 80% correlation was noted in samples from AIDS and ARC patients in Scandinavia (4,36,37), Switzerland (70), Italy (our personal observation), France (43), Great Britain (9) and Australia (14). In addition, serum antibodies to HTLV-III have been detected in a high percentage of AIDS patients from Africa (6). This was also true for a high proportion of the normal population in many areas of Africa, including sera sampled in 1972-1973 (68). These observations, coupled with the finding of antibody to HTLV-I and occasionally infectious virus (23,28,67,81) in many specimens of old world primates, are consistent with the hypothesis that the HTLV viruses originated in Africa. It is clear that seropositivity indicates that virus most likely can be isolated from the person's lymphocytes (serum antibody means that active virus replication at some point in time). It is possible, however, that in some rare instances, e.g., hemophilia, individuals receiving multiple donations of blood products containing inactive virus or viral proteins may develop a purely immune response.

HTLV-III PROTEINS

The protein profile of sucrose-density banded HTLV-III virions is similar to that of HTLV-I and HTLV-II. Major viral, Comassie Blue, stained, bands of disrupted HTLV-III supplemented by have molecular weights 40,000-46,000, 24,000 and 15,000-17,000 daltons. These proteins are believed to correspond to the envelope glycoprotein and the major <u>gag</u> proteins of the virus. A comparison of the antigenic properties of HTLV-III with those of HTLV-I and HTLV-II using the Western blot analysis also demonstrated some antigenic cross-reactivity (our personal observation). The results of those tests looking specifically at cross-reactivities in p24 antigens among all of these viruses can be summarized as: 1) A strong antibody reaction with the homologous proteins. 2) Moderate reactivities between HTLV-I p24 and antibody to HTLV-II and between HTLV-III p24 and antibody to HTLV-II. 3) Weak reactions between HTLV-I p24 and antibody to HTLV-III. This indicates that a specific, although distant, homology exists between the viruses studies. As will be discussed below, nucleotide sequence analysis confirms that some homology exists between the 3 HTLV's, especially the gag-pol region of the genome (2,55).

Competition radioimmunoassays of HTLV-III p24 also demonstrated that HTLV-III is a unique retrovirus whose major core protein, p24, is distinct from other animal retroviruses (69, and our personal observation). Consistent with Western blot analysis, these procedures also revealed a low but detectable level of antigenic cross-reactivity between HTLV-III and HTLV-I and HTLV-II (not shown). These cross-reactivities are, however, seen more clearly by Western blot analysis analogous to the detection of cross-reactivities between HTLV-I p24 and bovine leukemia virus (BLV) p24 by the Western blot procedures (50).

MOLECULAR BIOLOGY OF HTLV-III

Molecular Cloning and Analysis of the HTLV-III Genome. Once HTLV-III had been isolated and produced in sufficient quantities, the molecular cloning and analysis of its genome was undertaken. The H9/HTLV-III cell line (54) was used as the source of virus from which to clone the AIDS agent, since it was the source of viral reagents for all of the previous seroepidemiological studies of HTLV-III in AIDS. Lambda phage libraries were prepared from low molecular weight (Hirt) DNA of acutely infected H9 cells and from H9/HTLV-III chromosomal DNA containing the integrated HTLV-III provirus as described (25,71,72). These two libraries were then probed with ^{32}P-cDNA prepared from density gradient-purified virus from the H9/HTLV-III cell line. Figure 4 illustrates two full-length proviral clones, λHXB-2 and λHXB-3, and two nearly complete clones of the replicative intermediate form of HTLV-III (λBH-10 and λBH-5/8). The overall length of the HTLV-III provirus was found to be approximately 10 kb. Identical restriction patterns (Bgl II - Sst I - Hind III) spaced approximately 9 kb apart in each of the two proviral clones (λHXB-2 and λHXB-3) were noted and subsequently proven to represent the viral long terminal repeat (LTR) elements. In order to demonstrate that the restriction site cleavage pattern of the viral clones was an accurate representation of the HTLV-III genome, DNA from virally-infected H9 cells was digested with various enzymes and blot hybridized to a molecular probe derived from the λBH-10 clone. The restriction fragments predicted from maps of the viral clones were found experimentally by Southern analysis (data not shown). Furthermore, while the HTLV-III probe λBH-10 hybridized well to HTLV-III infected DNA, it did not hybridize to uninfected DNA including uninfected H9 cells, uninfected HT cells (the parent cell line from which H9 was cloned), or other normal human DNAs (data not shown). These data indiate that HTLV-III, like HTLV-I and HTLV-II, is an exogenous retrovirus lacking nucleic acid sequences derived from human DNA.

Using the cloned probes for HTLV-III, the characteristics of viral integration in cell lines and fresh tissues infected with HTLV-III were examined. It was found that HTLV-III, unlike most other retroviruses, persists in chronically-infected cells as both integrated and unintegrated DNA. Since persistence of unintegrated viral DNA is an uncommon property for retroviruses, and since it has previously been associated with cytopathic properties, the possibility has been raised (25,72,73) that unintegrated HTLV-III DNA could be involved in the virus' cytopathic effects in vitro and in vivo as suggested in other systems (34,80).

The finding that the proviral form of HTLV-III is polyclonally integrated in chronically infected cell lines also distinguishes HTLV-III from HTLV-I and HTLV-II. These latter viruses have, in addition to a cytopathic effect on infected cells, a predominant transforming effect which leads to a monoclonally expanded population of cells. Since HTLV-III has not been shown to possess transforming properties, it is not surprising that even chronically infected cells contain polyclonally integrated provirus. However, it is not known whether this polyclonality is due to the continuous reinfection of neighboring cells or to the stable growth of a population of immortalized cells having HTLV-III integrated at random sites.

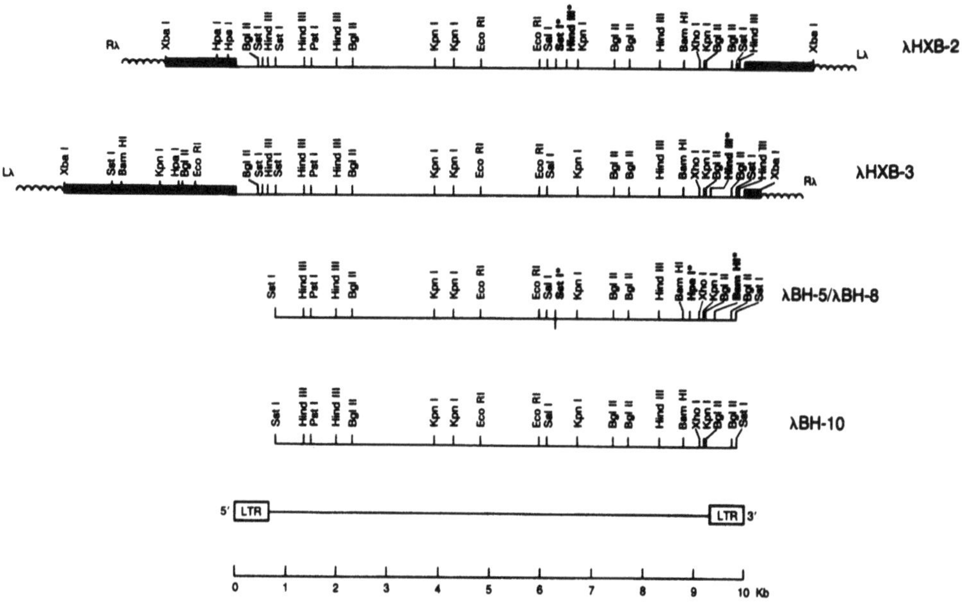

Figure 4. Restriction endonuclease maps of four closely related clones of HTLV-III. λHXB-2 and λHXB-3 represent full-length integrated proviral forms of HTLV-III. These clones contain the complete provirus (thin lines) including two LTR regions plus flanking cellular sequences (heavy lines). Clones λBH-10 and λBH-5/λBH-8 were derived from the linear unintegrated replicative intermediate form of HTLV-III in acutely infected H9 cells. It should be noted that λBH-5/λBH-8 consists of two separately cloned Sst I fragments (λBH-5 and λBH-8) which together compromise one HTLV-III genomic equivalent but which are not necessarily derived from the same viral molecule. Also, because λBH-10 and λBH-5 were cloned using the restriction enzyme Sst I, they lack 5' LTR sequences as shown. Other differences in the restriction maps between these HTLV-III clones are indicated by bold letters and asterisks, using λBH-10 as a reference (reproduced from reference 72 with permission).

The availability of the cloned HTLV-III genome also allowed a comparison of the sequence homology between HTLV-III and other retroviruses. The relatedness of HTLV-III to HTLV-I and -I and to gibbon ape leukemia virus (as a control) was initially compared, and distant but significant homology between HTLV-III and -II was found (2,71). These findings have now been confirmed by nucleotide sequence analysis of HTLV-III genome (55,63,78). Subsequently, in collaboration with M. Gonda and J. Clements, the relationship between HTLV-III and Visna virus, a virus which shares certain biologic properties with HTLV-III, was examined. These studies showed that HTLV-III is substantially more related to Visna virus at the nucleic acid level than it is to either HTLV-I or -II (20).

Genomic Diversity of HTLV-III

An analysis of molecular clones derived from the H9/HTLV-III cell line demonstrated that several distinguishable but highly related forms of the HTLV-III virus were present. Since this cell line had originally been infected with virus isolates from different AIDS or ARC patients, the possibility was raised whether the HTLV-III genome might differ from one isolate to another, or from one geographic region to another. To study this question, the restriction maps of different HTLV-III isolates obtained from individual patients whose clinical histories were well known were analyzed. An example of these genomic variations in several isolates of HTLV-III compared by Southern blot analysis with two restriction endonucleases is shown in Figure 5. In addition to a variaton seen with cells infected by the different HTLV-III isolates, this same variation was observed using DLH extracted from fresh patient cells. A detailed comparison of the restriction pattern of one of the most divergent isolates of HTLV-III obtained from a Haitian man (R.F.) with AIDS to those in the H9/HTLV-III cell line demonstrated that the provirus from R.F. contained two Sst I sites, presumably in the LTR regions, which generated a 9 kb fragment indistinguishable in size from that in H9/HTLV-III, λHXB-3, or λBH-10. However, the HTLV-III virus R.F. was substantially different from the predominant viral forms in H9/HTLV-III in most other restriction sites including EcoRI, Hind III, Bgl I, and Pst I. Further analysis of the full-length viral genome of $HTLV\text{-}III_{RF}$ revealed a difference in at least 16 out of 32 restriction sites. Moreover, heteroduplex analysis demonstrated that this divergence from the H9/HTLV-III clones occurred primarily in the 3' third of the genome where the envelope gene is known to exist (data not shown). These findings thus demonstrate that the genomes of different HTLV-III isolates may vary substantially.

To date, approximately 30 isolates of HTLV-III have been examined by restriction mapping and a spectrum of diversity ranging from isolates which are quite similar in the majority of restriction sites mapped to others which differ considerably, such as isolate $HTLV\text{-}III_{RF}$ described above were found. The reason for the diversity in the genomic restriction maps of different HTLV-III isolates is not known but could simply be a result of the highly replicative nature of this virus as suggested for another virus (49). Alternatively, some differences could reflect biological, temporal or geographical differences among the viruses.

Nucleotide Sequence Analysis of HTLV-III and Demonstration of Trans-Activation of the HTLV-III TR Elements

In collaboration with W. Haseltine, M. Pearson, and others, the complete nucleotide sequence of HTLV-III was recently determined in this laboratory (55) and by others (63,78). Like other retroviruses, HTLV-III was found to have 5' open reading frames encoding *gag* and *pol* proteins. The structure of the 3' half of the virus was unusual in that it contained two open reading frames: a 203 amino acid frame overlapping with the 3' end of the *pol* gene, and a longer open reading frame of 863 amino acids 3' to this first sequence. The function of this short open reading frame is unknown, but it may represent a noncoding vestigial *env* gene. The long open reading frame is thought to encode two functional polypeptides, a precursor of the envelope glycoprotein and an additional protein analogous to the *lor* product of HTLV-I, HTLV-II, and BLV. In this regard, it is important that the LTR of HTLV-III has recently been shown to be transcriptionally activated in virally infected cells, presumably by a product of its *lor* gene, as has been shown to occur with HTLV-I, HTLV-II, and BLV.

Because HTLV-I, HTLV-II, HTLV-III, BLV, and Visna virus share structural and functional properties, including a lor gene, trans-activation of their LTRs, varying degrees of nucleic acid homology, as well as certain biological functions (27,35,40,75,76), it is believed that these viruses are evolutionarily related.

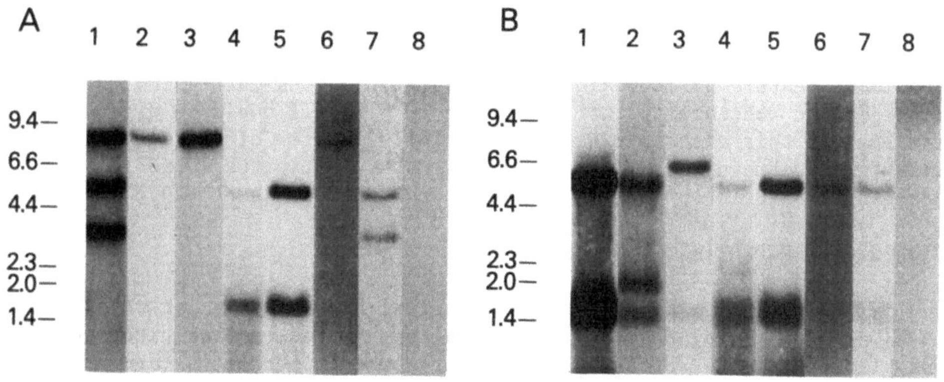

Figure 5. Demonstration of genomic variation in seven isolates of HTLV-III by Southern blot analysis. Panel A - Sst I. Panel B - Bgl II. DNA was obtained from the H9/HTLV-III line (lane 1); from infected cell lines derived from a healthy HTLV-III carrier (lane 2); a man with AIDS (lane 3); a man with ARC (lane 4); and a child with ARC (lane 5); from a biopsied lymph node of a man with AIDS (lane 6); from a cell line infected with virus from a man with ARC (lane 7); and from normal uninfected peripheral blood lymphocytes.

Detection of HTLV-III DNA in Fresh Tissues From AIDS and ARC Patients.

In order to obtain further insight into the tissue distribution of HTLV-III, a variety of fresh tissue specimens from 79 patients with ARC or AIDS were examined for the presence of HTLV-III DNA by Southern hybridization using cloned viral probes. HTLV-III sequences were detected in only 14 of the 79 patients evaluated. Viral sequences were most commonly found in lymph node, spleen, and brain, and only rarely in peripheral blood cells, and in none of seven Kaposi's sarcoma tissue specimens examined. It appears from these observations that only a minor population of cells in the tissues examined are infected with HTLV-III. This is apparent since virus can be routinely isolated from lymphocytes derived from these tissues by cell culture techniques, whereas viral DNA sequences are detected by Southern hybridization only infrequently. This observation was also confirmed by in situ hybridization where only a very low number of cells expressing viral RNA were detected (our personal observation with M. Harper).

The observations made here could have important implications regarding some of the clinical manifestations associated with the development of AIDS. For example, the lymph node enlargement commonly found in ARC patients would not appear to be a result of the proliferation of only HTLV-III-infected cells. The same conclusion is also likely for Kaposi's sarcoma since Kaposi's specimens examined in this study had been estimated by histopathologic examination to contain greater than 30 percent Kaposi's sarcoma (K.S.) cells. We found no evidence for HTLV-III viral DNA in any of the K.S. tumor specimens, and thus HTLV-III must be only indirectly involved in the pathogenesis of the characteristic skin tumors.

A possibly very important finding made in this fresh tissue survey was the detection of HTLV-III proviral DNA in cells from the brains of some AIDS cases (73). Unexplained central nervous system dysfunction, frequently manifest as dementia, or AIDS encephalopathy, constitutes a prominent feature of many AIDS cases (13,74). It is intriguing to consider the possibility that infection by HTLV-III could be directly involved in this disease process, especially in view of the many similarities found between HTLV-II and Visna virus, a lentivirus noted for pathologic effects on the central nervous system of sheep (20).

BIOLOGICAL PROPERTIES OF HTLV-III

Virus isolation and seroepidemiological data clearly linked HTLV-III to AIDS, and a study of other biological properties of this virus further established this correlation. When introduced into cell culture fresh mononuclear lymphocytes from AIDS, ARC, and asymptomatic donors at risk for AIDS usually released virus within 2-3 weeks. As illustrated in Figure 1, during this time period a significant loss of viable cells, predominantly those with the OKT4/ Leu 3a (helper/inducer) phenotype, was also observed. Also, when HTLV-III was used to infect fresh human mononuclear cells from normal donors virus was released (usually within 1-2 weeks following infection), many multinucleated giant cells were formed, and viable cells were lost (usually complete by 2-3 weeks in cell culture occurs). This cytopathic effect was even more rapid and dramatic when T-cells enriched for OKT4/ Leu3a+ markers were used. In this instance, the infected OKT4/leu3a+ population rapidly released virus and died within the first several days in cell culture. Many of the in vitro characteristics of HTLV-III-infected cells are, therefore, similar to the pathological picture observed in vivo. Other cell type populations such as OKT8/leu2a and non-T cells, however, when treated in the same way remained in cell culture for many weeks. There was some indication that cells other than those with the OKT4/ leu 3+ phenotypes can be infected by HTLV-III, e.g., B-lymphocytic cells and monocytoid cells (our personal observation). It is conceivable that these cells could be involved as a natural reservoir of virus in vivo.

HTLV INFECTION OF ESTABLISHED CELL LINES

Many established cell lines were also tested as possible targets for HTLV-III infection. As was described previously (54), one neoplastic aneuploid T-cell line derived from an adult with lymphoid leukemia and termed HT was found to be susceptible to infection with HTLV-III and, after single cell clones were infected, some were found to constitutively produce virus. This represented a major step in the study of AIDS since, for the first time, large amounts of virus could be produced for the preparation of immunological reagents and nucleic acid.

In addition to HT and its subclones, human T or pre-T cell lines (e.g., JM, CEM-CCRF, Molt 3,) were found permissive for infection infected by and production of HTLV-III (53, and our personal observations).

Furthermore, some B-lymphoblastic cell lines can also be productively infected by HTLV-III (47, and our personal observation). The cytopathic effect of HTLV-III described with fresh lymphocytes is also observed with T- and B-cell lines, although in some instances it was not as pronounced, since cells in some populations could survive and continue to produce virus. Cell lines with monocyte/macrophage characteristics can also be infected by HTLV-III (our personal observations). However, in contrast to the cytopathic effect seen with T and B lymphocytes, little or no virus-related cell death was observed. This again suggests the possibility that cells other than T-lymphocytes could also be infected in vivo and serve as a reservoir for virus in vivo. These established cell lines should prove very useful, not only as a source of large amounts of virus, but conceivably as a model system to study of cytopathic effect of HTLV-III on susceptible cells.

HTLV-III INFECTION OF NON-HUMAN PRIMATES

A recent report has also indicated subhuman primates, i.e. chimpanzees, can be infected by HTLV-III. In addition to an immunological response, i.e., production of virus specific antibody, and the ability to isolate virus from peripheral blood lymphocytes, clinical manifestations including lymphadenopathy similar to those seen in human patients were observed (1).

CYTOPATHIC EFFECT OF HTLV-III

The mechanisms responsible for the cytopathic effect of HTLV-III on infected cells, particularly those with the OKT4/leu 3a phenotype, are not known. Studies of virus-cell interactions have shown that the reason for the preferential tropism of HTLV-III for helper/inducer T-cells is that the receptor for virus infection on the cell surface cross reacts with, if not identical to, the antigens (T4) detected by monoclonal antibody OKT4/ leu 3a, and others (10,53). It has been suggested that HTLV-III infected cells liberate potent immunoregulatory factors which suppress the function of T- and other cells of the immune system (38) and our preliminary experience with T cells infected by HTLV-III in vitro supports this observation. Supernatant fluids from fresh cultured human mononuclear leukocytes infected with HTLV-III contain activities able to suppress the activation of both T- and B-cell (Markham et al., in preparation). The significance of these observations and how, or if, these activities differ from those obtained from stimulated normal T cells remain to be elucidated.

BIOLOGICAL COMPARISONS OF HTLV-I, -II AND -III

As discussed previously, other members of the HTLV family of retroviruses, i.e., HTLV-I and II, also infect fresh human T lymphocytes. However, several differences between the effect of HTLV-III and the previously isolated viruses were noted, the obvious difference being the well defined transformation of human T lymphocytes by HTLV-I and II. No evidence for the transformation of infected cells by HTLV-III has been obtained, to date. In addition, other biological differences included: 1) transmission of HTLV-III to fresh human lymphocytes was most efficient using cell-free virus whereas HTLV-I usually required cocultivation procedures, 2) HTLV-III, like HTLV-I, can infect cord blood and bone marrow lymphocytes, but in addition HTLV-III readily infects normal adult peripheral blood lymphocytes which was accomplished with some difficulty with HTLV-I. This likely reflects a difference in the amount of virus produced (HTLV being a virus producer), and possibly in the concentration of target cells, and3) the primary targets of HTLV-I, -II and HTLV-III are OKT4/leu 3+ T-cells; however, the dramatic cytopathic effect observed with HTLV-III, although present, is not as evident with HTLV-I and -II infected cells.

Despite certain biological differences between HTLV-I, -II and -III, several observations, as described previously, suggested that all members of the HTLV family could exert an immunosuppressive effect on infected cells in vitro (reviewed in 44,45,52) and possibly in vivo (11). Furthermore, HTLV-I transformed cells were found to be a rich source of many immunoregulatory activities including: macrophage migration enhancing factor; leukocyte migration inhibitory factor; migration enhancing factor; macrophage activating factor; differentiation inducing activity; colony stimulating factor; eosinophil growth and maturation activity; fibroblast activating factor; and gamma interferon (60). Whether or not HTLV-III infected lymphocytes will also release these activators is under investigation. Although it was noted that cells (lymphoid and/or monocytoid cells) obtained from AIDS patients release factors that inhibit T and B cell function. Infection of normal leukocytes in vitro has extended these observations. Following infection of mononuclear cells from normal donor potent inhibition of T-cell activation by mitogens and of B-cell maturation were detected (our unpublished observation). It is not clear, however, whether these activities are unique to infection by HTLV-III, or are an elevated expression of normal activities, possibly enhanced by a trans-activation mechanism (described above).

CONTROL OF HTLV

The numbers of individuals suffering from diseases caused by HTLV-III have increased at an alarming rate during the previous 3 to 4 years. As discussed previously, individuals infected by the virus are no longer limited to a restricted population in the U.S., but now involve people with any one of several risk factors, and is spreading to other parts of the world. Two aspects of the control of HTLV-III (and its diseases) that need careful investigation are treatment of already infected individuals and prevention of further spread of infection. Possibly the most likely approaches for the treatment of infected people will be to find ways to: 1) inhibit virus infection or replication, 2) remove infected cells, including those possibly serving as a virus reservoir, and 3) replace lost T-lymphocytes. Procedures for the replacement of T-lymphocytes are by transplantation or by treatment with TCGF, are now well tested; however, procedures to control HTLV-III infection and replication, and for the removal of infected cells, remain to be developed. In this regard, certain drugs which were found to inhibit viral reverse transcriptase activity, e.g., Suramin, are promising candicates since they inhibit virus infection in vitro (46, and Resnick et al., in preparation). The preparation of vaccines to prevent infection is being actively pursued by different approaches in several laboratories. It is important to determine, however, if the genomic diversity among many HTLV-III isolates affects their antigenic composition. If this is the case, use of neutralizing sera would be less likely to have broad application. Low titers of neutralizing antibodies to HTLV-III have been detected in the serum of some infected individuals including patients who have developed disease (our personal observation with M. Robert-Guroff, R. Weiss et al. and M. Hirsch et al.). In these instances, the viral neutralizing activity was found to be associated with the immunoglobulin fraction of serum, and the same immunoglobulins recognized HTLV-III surface proteins. Although these observations need to be extended, it is encouraging that sera from many different patients and at-risk donors can affect one source of HTLV-III. It remains to be determined if this will be true for many different virus isolates.

SUMMARY

The newly identified human HTLV-III virus, the etiologic agent for AIDS, shares many of the biological and physicochemical properties common to a family of retroviruses named human T-cell leukemia (lymphotropic) viruses, or HTLV. Because of the similarities, and because of the uniform nomenclature for human T-cell leukemia (lymphotropic) viruses adopted at the first Cold Spring Harbor Meeting on HTLV (19,79), this newly discovered virus associated with AIDS as HTLV-III was named HTLV-III. Other investigators making independent isolations of virus have suggested naming the virus lymphadenopathy virus or LAV (3,16), immunodeficiency associated virus or IADV (48), AIDS-related virus (41). Immunological and nucleic acid comparison has now demonstrated that these viruses are, not surprisingly, very similar to HTLV-III (55,63,78). In view of the wide range of disease manifestations caused by the virus, and previous discussions concerning a uniform nomenclature for human T-lymphotropic retroviruses, it would seen ill-advised to restrict the name of this virus to one clinical manifestation of one disease.

The frequent isolation of HTLV-III from patients with AIDS and ARC, the detection of antibodies specific for HTLV-III in nearly all patients with these diseases and in a high proportion of individuals at risk, and finally its effect on cells in vitro, leaves little doubt that HTLV-III is causatively involved in the development of these diseases. This etiologic association is further strengthened by the detection of HTLV-III infection in many instances where a direct cause-and-effect association can be made, e.g., hemophiliacs and children with AIDS, and blood from HTLV-III infected donors and the otherwise normal recipients of this blood who subsequently develop AIDS.

Although the basic characterization of HTLV-III as a new retrovirus is now complete, there are many questions concerning its biological and biochemical properties which remain to be answered, including the fundamental question as to how the virus exerts its cytopathic effects and causes AIDS. The nucleotide sequence analysis of HTLV-III is now providing important information concerning the structural-functional relationships of the viral genome. This information, along with expression studies and analyses of viral-specific proteins, will be important to ongoing efforts to control viral infection and expression. One of the major observations resulting from these molecular studies is the identification of gene lor which likely codes for a trans-activating protein similar to that previously reported for HTLV-I and -II, and at least some members of the Lentivirus group, e.g., Visna virus (20). Also HTLV-III was found to share more genomic homology with Visna virus than with HTLV-I or -II. This suggests that a regrouping of the several mammalian retroviruses including the HTLV group and Lentivirus might be advisable.

The rapid spread of HTLV-III and the consequential diseases makes a rapid and thorough effort to control the virus imperative. Success has been reported with some drugs in vitro, and these need to be expanded. A determining factor relevant to the development of effective vaccines against these viruses will be whether the genomic diversity found among virus isolates are of biological or immunological significance. The availability of many isolates of HTLV-III from donors having various disease manifestations, and from different geographic areas, along with the ability to grow HTLV-III in large quantities, and the availability of genomic clones, should provide the reagents needed to address these questions. Such studies involving patients with AIDS and ARC, as well as apparently healthy carriers, will undoubtedly lead in the near future to a more complete understanding of HTLV-III and the disease(s) it produces.

ACKNOWLEDGEMENT

We wish to acknowledg the contributions of M. Popovic, F. Wong-Staal, S. Arya, S. Josephs, L. Ratner, M. Robert-Guroff, and C. Saxinger for contribution of scientific information, and to many clinical collaborators for the provision of valuable patient materials.

REFERENCES

1. Alter, H.J., Eichberg, J.W., Masur, H., et al., Transmission of HTLV-III Infection from human plasma to chimpanzees: An animal model for AIDS, Science, 226:549-552 (1984).
2. Arya, S.K., Gallo, R.C., Hahn, B.H. et al., Homology of genomes of AIDS-associated virus with genomes of human T-cell leukemia viruses, Science, 225:927-930 (1984).
3. Barré-Sinoussi, F., Chermann, J.C., Rey, F., Nugeyne, M.T., Chamaret, S., Gruest, J., Dauguet, C., Axler-Blin, C., Vezinet-Brun, F., Rouzioux, C., Rozenbaum, W., and Montagnier, L., Isolation of a T-lymphotropic retrovirus from a patient at risk for acquired immune deficiency syndrome (AIDS), Science, 220:868-871 (1983).
4. Bieberfeld, G., Bredberg-Ruden, U., Battiger, B., et al., Antibodies to human T-lymphotropic virus (HTLV) type-III demonstrated by a dot immunobinding assay, Scand. J. Immunol., in press.
5. Broder, S., Gallo, R.C., A pathogenic retrovirus (HTLV-III) linked to AIDS, N. Engl. J. Med., 311:1292-1297 (1984).
6. Brun-Vezinet, F., Rouzioux C., Montagnier, L., et al., Prevalence of antibodies to lymphadenopathy-associated retrovirus in African patients with AIDS, Science, 226:453-456 (1984).
7. Centers for Disease Control Task Force on Kaposi's Sarcoma and Opportunistic Infections, Epidemiological aspects of the current outbreak of Kaposi's sarcoma and opportunistic infections, N. Engl. J. Med., 306:248-252 (1982).
8. Clumeck, N., Sonnett, J., Taelman, H., Acquired Immunodeficiency Syndrome in African Patients, N. Engl. J. Med., 310:492-497 (1984).
9. Cheingson-Popov, R., Weiss, R.A., Dalgleish, A., et al., Prevalence of antibody to HTLV-III in AIDS and AIDS-risk patients in Britain, The Lancet, i:477-480 (1984).
10. Dalgliesh, H.G., Beverly, P.C.L., Clapham, M., et al., The CD4 (T4) antigen is an essential component of the receptor for the AIDS retrovirus, Nature, 312:763-767 (1984).
11. Essex, M., McLane, M.F., Lee, T.H., Falk, L., Howe, C.W.S., Mullins, J.I., Cabradilla, C., and Francis, D.P., Antibodies to cell membrane antigens associated with human T-cell leukemia virus in patients with AIDS, Science, 220:859-862 (1983).
12. Essex, M.E., McLane, M.F., Tachibana, N., Francis, D.P., and Lee, T.-H., Seroepidemiology of human T-cell leukemia virus in relation to immunosuppression and the acquired immunodeficiency syndrome, in: "Human T-Cell Leukemia/Lymphoma Virus", R.C. Gallo, M. Essex and L. Gross, eds., Cold Spring Harbor Laboratory, New York, (1984).
13. Epstein, L.G., Sharer, L.R., Joshi, V.V. et al., Progressive encephalopathy in children with AIDS, Ann. Neurol,. (in press).
14. Frazer, I.H., Sarngadharan, M.G., Mackay, J.R., et al., Antibody to human T-cell leukemia virus Type-III in Australian homosexual men with lymphadenopathy, The Medical J. of Australia, 141:224-226 (1984).
15. Fauci, A.S., Macher, A.M., Longo, D.L., et al., Acquired immunodeficiency syndrome: epidemiological, clinical, immunologic and therapeutic considerations, Ann. Intern. Med., 160:92-106 (1984).
16. Feorino, P.M., Kalyanaraman, V.S., Haverkos, H.W., et al., Lymphadenopathy associated virus infection of a blood donor-recipient pair with acquired immunodeficiency syndrome, Science, 225:69-72 (1984).

17. Gallo, R.C., Human T-cell leukemia-lymphoma virus and T-cell malignancies in adults, in: "Cancer Surveys", L.M. Franks, J. Wyke, and R.A. Weiss, eds., Vol. 3, Oxford University Press, Oxford (1984).
18. Gallo, R.C., Salahuddin, S.Z., Popovic, M., Shearer, G.M., Kaplan, M., Haynes, B.F., Palker, T.J., Redfield, R., Oleske, J., Safai, B., White, F., Foster, P., and Markham, P.D., Frequent Detection and Isolation of Cytopathic Retroviruses (HTLV-III) from Patients with AIDS and at risk for AIDS, Science, 224:500-503 (1984).
19. Gallo, R.C., Essex, M., and Gross, L., eds., "Human T-Cell Leukemia/Lymphoma Virus", Cold Spring Harbor Press, New York, 1984.
20. Gonda, M.A., Wong-Staal, F., Gallo, R.C., et al., Sequence homology and morphologic similarity of HTLV-III and visna virus, a pathogenic lentivirus, Science, 227:173-177 (1985).
21. Groopman, J.E., Salahuddin, S.Z., Sarngadharan, M.G., Markham, P.D., Gonda, M., Sliski, A., Gallo, R.C., Isolation of HTLV-III from saliva of pre-AIDS, AIDS and healthy homosexual men at risk for AIDS, Science, 226:447-449 (1984).
22. Guinan, M.E., Thomas, P.A., Pinsky, P.F., et al., Heterosexual and homosexual patients with the acquired immunodeficiency syndrome, Ann Intern. Med., 100:213-8 (1984).
23. Guo, H.G., Wong-Staal, F., Gallo, R.C., Novel viral sequences related to a human T-cell leukemia virus in T-cells of a seropositive baboon, Science, 223:1195-1197 (1984).
24. Hahn, B.H., Shaw, G.M., Popovic, M., et al., Molecular cloning and analysis of a new variant of human T-cell leukemia virus (HTLVIb) from an African patient with adult T-cell leukemia-lymphoma, Int. J. Cancer, 34:613-618 (1984).
25. Hahn, B.H., Shaw, G.M., Arya, S.K., et al., Molecular cloning and characterization of the virus associated with AIDS (HTLV-III), Nature, 312:166-169 (1984).
26. Harris, C., Small, C.B., Klein, R.E., et al., Immunodeficiency in female sexual partners of men with the acquired immunodeficiency syndrome, N. Engl. J. Med., 308:1181-4 (1983).
27. Haseltine, W.A., Sodroski, J., Patarca, R., et al., Structure of 3' terminal region of type II human T lymphotropic virus: Evidence for new coding region Science, 225:419-421 (1984).
28. Hayami, M., Komuro, A., Nozawa, K., et al., Prevalence of antibody to adult T-cell leukemia virus-associated antigen (ATLVA) in Japanese monkeys and other non-human primates, Int. J. Cancer, 33:179-183 (1984).
29. Hirsch, M.S., Wormser, C.P., Schooley, R.T., et al., Risk of nosocomial infection with human T-cell lymphotropic virus III (HTLV-III), N. Engl. J. Med., 312:1-4 (1985).
30. Ho, D.B., Schooling, R.T., Rota, T.R., Kaplan, J.C., Flyn, T., Salahuddin, Z., Gonda, M., and Hirsch, M.S., HTLV-III in the semen and blood of a healthy homosexual man, Science, 226:451-453 (1984).
31. Jaffe, A.N., Sarngadharan, M.G., Durco, A., et al., Serologic evidence of an etiologic role for a human T-lymphotropic retrovirus in transfusion-associated AIDS, Submitted.
32. Kalyanaraman, V.S., Sarngadharan, M.G., Bunn, P.A., Minna, J.D., and Gallo, R.C., Antibodies in human sera reactive against an internal structural protein of human T-cell lymphoma virus, Nature, 294:271-273 (1981).
33. Kalyanaraman, V.S., Sarngadharan, M.G., Robert-Gufoff, M., Miyoshi I, Blayney, D., Golde, D., and Gallo, R.C., A new subtype of human T-cell leukemia virus (HTLV-II) assocated with a T-cell varient of hairy cell leukemia, Science, 218:571-573 (1982).
34. Keshet, E. and Temin, H.M., Cell killing by spleen necrosis virus is correlated with a transcient accumulation of spleen necrosis virus DNA, J. Virol., 31:376-388 (1979).

35. Kiyokawa, T., Seiki, M., et al., Identification of a protein (p40) encoded by a 3'-OH sequence pX of human T-cell leukemia virus type-I, Gann, 25:247-251 (1984).
36. Krohn, K., Ranki, A., Antoner, J., et al., Immune functions in homosexual men with antibodies to HTLV-III in Finland, Clin. Exp. Immunol., in press.
37. Lange-Wantzin, C., Saxinger, W.C., Gallo, R.C., Prevalence of HTLV-III antibodies in Danish homosexuals with venereal disease, ACTA Dermat., (Stockholm), in press.
38. Lawrence, J., and Mayer, S., Immunoregulatory lymphokines of T-hybridomas from AIDS patients: constitutive and inducible suppressor factors, Science, 225:66-69 (1984).
39. Lee, T.H., Coligan, J.E., Homma, T., McLane, M.F., Tachibana, N., and Essex, M., Human T-cell leukemia virus-associated cell membrane antigens: Identity of the major antigens recognized by the virus infection, Proc. Natl. Acad. Sci. USA, 81:3856-3860.
40. Lee, T.H., Coligan, J.E., Sodroski, J.G., et al., Antigen encoded by the 3' terminal region of human T-cell leukemia virus: evidence for a functional gene, Science, 226:57-61 (1984).
41. Levy, J.A., Hoffman, A.D., Kramer, S.M., Landin, J.A., Shimabukuro, J.M., and Oshiro, L.S., Isolation of lymphocytopathic retroviruses from San Francisco patients with AIDS, Science, 225:840-842 (1984).
42. Markham, P.D., Salahuddin, S.Z., Veren, K., Orndorff, S., Gallo, R.C., Enhanced expression and isolation of HTLV-III using hydrocortisone and other hormones, Submitted, (1985).
43. Matherz, D., Leibowitch, J., Mathern, S., et al., Antibodies to HTLV-III in serum from AIDS and patients at risk for AIDS in France, Submitted.
44. Mitsuya, H., Guo, H.G., Megson, Me. et al., Transformation and cyto-pathogenic effect in an immune human T-cell clone infected by HTLV-I, Science, 223:1293-1296 (1984).
45. Mitsuya, H., Matis, L.A., Megson, M., Bunn, P.A., Murray, C., Mann, D.L., Gallo, R.C., and Broder, S., Generation of an HLA-restricted cytotoxic T-cell line reactive against cultured tumor cells from a patient infected with human T-cell leukemia/lymphoma virus, J. Exp. Med., 158:994-999 (1983).
46. Mitsuya, H., Popovic, M., Yarchoan, R., Matsushita, S., Gallo, R.C., Broder, S, Suramin protection of T-cells in vitro against infec-tivity and cytopathic effect of HTLV-III, Science, 226:172-174 (1984).
47. Montagnier, L., Grust, J., Chamaret, S., Daugnet, C., Axler, C., Guetard, D., Nugeyre, M.T., Barré-Sinoussi, F., Cherman, J.C., Brunet, J.B., Klatzmann, D., Glockman, J.C., Adaptation of lymph-adenopathy-associated virus (LAV) to replication in EBV-transformed, B-lymphoblastoid cells lines, Science, 225:63-66 (1984).
48. Montagnier, L., Chermann, J.C., Barré-Sinoussi, F., Chamaret, S., Gruest, J., Nugeyre, M.T., Rey, F., Dauguet, C., Axler-Blin, C., Vezinet-Brux, F., Rouzioux, C., Saimot, G.A., Rozenbaum, W., Gluckman, J.C., Klatzmann, D., Vilmer, E., Griscelli, C., Foyer-Gazengel, C., and Brunet, J.B., A new human T-lymphotropic retro-virus: characterization and possible role in lymphadenopathy and acquired immune deficiency syndrome, in: "Human T-cell leukemia (Lympoma Virus)", R.C. Gallo, M.E. Enox, and L. Gross, eds., Cold Spring Harbor Laboratories, (1984).
49. O'Rear, J.J., and Temin, H.M., Spontaneous changes in the nucleotide sequence in proviruses of spleen necrosis virus, an avian retrovirus, Proc. Natl. Acad. Sci., 79:1230-1234 (1982).
50. Oroszlan, S., Copeland, T.D., Kalyanaraman, V.S., et al., Chemical analysis of human T-cell leukemia virus structural proteins, in: "Human T-cell Leukemia/Lymphoma Virus, R.C. Gallo, M. Essex, L. Gross, eds., Cold Spring Harbor Laboratory, (1984).

51. Plot, P., Taelman, H., Minlangu, K.B., et al., Acquired immunodeficiency syndrome in a heterosexual population in Zaire., The Lancet, ii:65-69 (1984).
52. Popovic, M., Flomenberg, N., Volkman, D.J., Mann, D., Fauci, A.S., Dupont, B., and Gallo, R.C., Alteration of T-cell functions by infection with HTLV-I or HTLV-II, Science, 226:459-462 (1984).
53. Popovic, M., Read-Conade, E., Gallo, R.C., T4 positive human neoplastic cell lines susceptible to and permissive for HTLV-III, Lancet, ii:1473-1475 (1984).
54. Popovic, M., Sarngadharan, M.G., Reed, E., and Gallo, R.C., Detection, isolation, and continuous production of cytopathic human T lymphotropic retrovirus (HTLV-III) from patients with AIDS and pre-AIDS, Science, 224:497-500 (1984).
55. Ratner, L., Haseltine, W., Patarea, R., et al., Complete nucleotide sequence of AIDS virus, HTLV-III, Nature, 313:277-284 (1985).
56. Redfield, R., Markham, P.D., Salahuddin, S.Z., et al., Frequent transmission of HTLV-III among spouses of patients with AIDS-related complex (ARC) and the acquired immune deficiency syndrome AIDS: A family study, J. Am. Med. Assoc., In press (1985).
57. Robert-Guroff, M. and Gallo, R.C., Establishment of an etiologic relationship between the human T-cell leukemia/lymphoma virus (HTLV) and adult T-cell leukemia, Blüt,:1-12 (1983).
58. Robert-Guroff, M., Safai, B., Gelmann, E., et al., HTLV-I specific antibody in AIDS patients and others at risk, Lancet, ii:128-131 (1984).
59. Safai, B., Sarngadharan, M.G., Groopman, J.E., et al., Seroepidemiological studies of HTLV-III in AIDS, Lancet, 1:1438-1440 (1984).
60. Salahuddin, S.Z., Markham, P.D., Lindner, S.G., Gootenberg, J., Popovic, M., Hemmi, H., Sarin, P.S., and Gallo, R.C., Lymphokine production by cultured human T-cells transformed by human T-cell leukemia-lymphoma virus, Science, 223:703-706 (1984).
61. Salahuddin, S.Z., Groopman, J., Markham, P.D., et al., HTLV-III in symptom-free seronegative persons, The Lancet, ii:1418-1420 (1984).
62. Salahuddin, S.Z., Markham, P.D., Popovic, M., Sarngadharan, M.G., Orndorff, S., Pladager, A., Patel, A., Gold, J., Gallo, R.C., One hundred-and-one infectious HTLV-III isolates from AIDS and ARC patients and clinically normal donors at risk for AIDS, Proc. Natl. Acad. Sci. USA, Submitted (1985).
63. Sanchez-Pescador, R., Power, M.D., Barr, P.J., et al., Nucleotide sequence and expression of an AIDS-associated retrovirus (ARV-2), Science, 227:484-492 (1985).
64. Sarngadharan, M.G., Alludeen, H.S., and Gallo, R.C., Reverse transcriptase of RNA tumor viruses and animal cells, Method. Cancer Res., 12:3-47 (1976).
65. Sarngadharan, M.G., Popovic, M., Bruch, L., Schüpbach, J., Gallo, R.C., Antibodies reactive with a human T lymphotropic retrovirus (HTLV-III) in the sera of patients with acquired immune deficiency syndrome, Science, 224:506-508 (1983).
66. Saxinger, W.C., Blattner, W.A., Levine, P.H., Clark, J., Biggar, R., Hoh, M., Moghissi, J., Jacobs, P., Wilson, L., Jacobson, T., Crookes, R., Strong, M., Ansari, A.A., Dean, A.G., Nkrumah, R.K., Mourali, N., and Gallo, R.C., Human T-cell leukemia virus (HTLV-I) antibodies in Africa, Science, 225:1473-1476 (1984).
67. Saxinger, W.X., Lange-Wentzin, G., Thomsen, K., et al., Human T-cell leukemia virus: A disease family of related exogenous retroviruses of humans and Old World primates, in:"Human T-Cell Leukemia/Lymphoma Virus", R.C. Gallo, M. Essex, L. Gross, eds., Cold Spring Harbor Laboratory, NY. (1984).
68. Saxinger, W.C., Levine, P.H., Dean, A.G., et al., Evidence for exposure to HTLV-III in Uganda prior to 1973, Science, in press (1985).

69. Schüpbach, J., Sarngadharan, M.G. and Gallo, R.C., Antigens on HTLV-infected cells recognized by leukemia and AIDS sera are related to HTLV viral glycoprotein, Science, 224:607-610 (1984).
70. Schüpbach, J., Haller, D., Vogt, M., et al., Antbodies to HTLV-III in Swiss patients with AIDS and pre-AIDS and in groups at risk for AIDS, N. Engl. J. Med., in press, (1985).
71. Shaw, G.M., Gonda, M.A., Flickenger, G.H., et al., Genomes of evolutionarily divergent members of the HTLV family are highly conserved especially in pX, Proc. Natl. Acad. Sci., 81:4544-4548 (1984).
72. Shaw, G.M., Hahn, B.H., Arya, S.K., et al., Molecular characterization of HTLV-III in AIDS, Science, 226:1165-1171 (1984).
73. Shaw, G.M., Harper, M.E., Hahn, B., et al., HTLV-III infection in brains of children and adults with AIDS encephalopathy, Science, 227:177-182 (1985).
74. Snider, W.D., Simpson, D.M., Nielson, S., et al., Neuroogic complication of AIDS: Analysis of 50 patients, Ann. Neurol., 14:403-418 (1983).
75. Sodroski, J., Rosen, C.A. and Haseltine, W.A., Trans-acting transcriptional activation of the long terminal repeat of HTLV in infected cells, Science, 225:381-385 (1984).
76. Sodroski, J., Posner, C., Wong-Staal, F., et al., Trans-acting transcriptional regulation of human T-cell leukemia virus type-III long terminal repeat, Science, 227:171-173 (1984).
77. Van de Pere, P., Lepage, P., Kostelyn, P., et al., Acquired immunodeficiency syndrome in Rwanda, The Lancet, ii:62-65 (1984).
78. Wain-Hobson, F., Sonigo, P., Danos, D., et al., Nucleotide seuquence of the AIDS virus, LAV, Cell, 40:9-17 (1985).
79. Watanabe, T., Seiki, M., and Yoshida M., Retrovirus terminology, Science, 222:1178 (1983).
80. Weller, S.K., Joy, A.E., and Temin, H.M., Correlation obetween cell killing and massive second-round superinfection by members of some subgroups of Avian Leukosis Virus, J. Virol., 33:494-506 (1980).
81. Yamamoto, N., Kobayashi, N., Takouchi, K., et al., Characterization of African green monkey B-cell lines releasing an adult T-cell leukemia virus-related agent, Int. J. Cancer, 34:77-82 (1984).
82. Zagury, D. Bernard, J., Leibowitch, J., Safai, B., Groopman, J.E., Veldman, M., Sarngadharan, Gallo, R.C., HTLV-III in cells cultured from semen of two patients with AIDS, Science, 226:449-451 (1984).

LYMPHADENOPATHY ASSOCIATED VIRUS (L.A.V.) : ITS ASSOCIATION WITH AIDS OR PRODROMES

Françoise Barré-Sinoussi and Jean-Claude Chermann

Unité d'Oncologie Virale, Institut Pasteur, 25 Rue du Dr. Roux, 75724 Paris Cédex 15, France

INTRODUCTION

In testing the hypothesis that retroviruses could be involved in AIDS or AIDS related complexe (ARC), we isolated in 1983 a T lymphotropic retrovirus from a homosexual man presenting with lymphadenopathy (1). This virus was shown to be a retrovirus by all classical criteria (density in sucrose gradient, high molecular weight RNA, reverse transcriptase activity, morphogenesis by budding) (2)(3). This first isolate was named Lymphadenopathy Associated Virus (LAV 1). Latter on similar viruses were obtained by our group (4)(5)(6) and by others from patients with AIDS or related symptoms (7)(8)(9).

Several other names were given such as IDAV, HTLV III or ARV, but all isolates were morphologically and antigenically similar to LAV 1 and clearly distinct from other known animal or human retroviruses such as HTLV I and HTLV II. The involvment of this new group is unanimously accepted. We summarize here the main characteristics of this novel type of human retrovirus and the data indicating why LAV is thought to be the primary agent of AIDS.

I. LAV isolates

LAV related viruses were obtained from all groups of patients having AIDS or at risk of AIDS according the method previously described (1). Briefly, lymphocytes from lymph node biopsies or from peripheral blood were stimulated with phytohemagglutinin (pHA) for three days and then cultured in the presence of T cell grown factor (TCGF) and antibodies to human interferon. The cells began to release virus particles from day 10 to day 25, as measured by reverse transcriptase activity in the cell free supernatant. As shown on table 1, 35 isolates were made from American and French homosexuals, hemophiliacs, Zairians, Haitians, American IV drug users, bone marrow transplants and a blood donor-recipient pair.

TABLE 1

GROUPS	DISEASE	Number of LAV isolates
Homosexuals	LAS AIDS	7 9
IV drug addicts	AIDS	4
Hemophiliacs	NO AIDS	1 1
Blood transfusion (a donor-recipient pair)	AIDS	2
Bone Marrow transplants	AIDS	2
Zairians	ARC AIDS	1 2
Haitians	LAS AIDS	3 2

Isolation was found to be easier from frank AIDS cases than from individuals with lymphadenopathy syndrome (LAS). In AIDS case, a failure in viral isolation was observed only when blood samples were obtained from patients at a very late stage of the disease.

In LAS, the virus was more easily isolated from lymphocytes derived from lymph node biopsies than from peripheral blood. This suggest that more lymphocytes express the virus in early diagnosed AIDS cases than in LAS patients.

One viral isolate was obtained from a healthy hemophiliac, brother of an hemophiliac with AIDS, (5) indicating the possible existence of asymptomatic virus carriers.

Heterosexual transmission was also suggested by virus isolation from a Zairian couple (6).

But in contrast, all attempts to isolate LAV from healthy blood donor or laboratory workers have failed.

II. Main characteristics of LAV isolates

All viral isolates have similar characteristics which can be summarized as followed :

1) Pecular morphology of LAV virions

Ultrathin sections of LAV producing lymphocytes showed budding particles on the cell surface with a thin dense crescent and typical mature particles with a small dense eccentric core. This morphology is clearly distinct from classical C type virions but ressembles to mature D type particles.

2) Tropism for T lymphocytes and cytopathic effect

We have previously demonstrated that only T4 lymphocytes were able to express the virus or to be infected by the virus (10). Recently D. Klatzmann and coll (11),as well as AG. Dalgleish and coll(12) have shown that the T 4 molecule itself may be the receptor for the virus.

Moreover, at the peak of virus production, an inhibition of cell proliferation was observed as well as a decrease of the T3 and T4 cell surface markers (1)(3). Giant multinucleated cells were also seen at the onset of virus production.(4)

These data indicated a cytopathic effect of the virus on target T cells.

3) LAV proteins

Previous studies on LAV proteins had revealed three major components p25, p18 and p13 in purified virions (3)(4). LAV p25 is a methionine rich ccmpound which is associated with the viral cores and represents the major core protein of the virus. LAV p25 is a highly conserved determinant since the major core proteins of different viral isolates are antigenically identical, but are not related to the major structural proteins of other animal or human retroviruses (4)(13).

The other two proteins (p18 and p13) are presumably also gag gene products.

All these proteins are antigenic in patients as demonstrated by radioimmunoprecipitation assay (4) or by Western Blot analysis (14). As shown on figure 1, sera from patients with AIDS or prodromes contain antibodies to LAV p25 and to LAV p18. In few cases antibodies to LAV p13 are also detected.

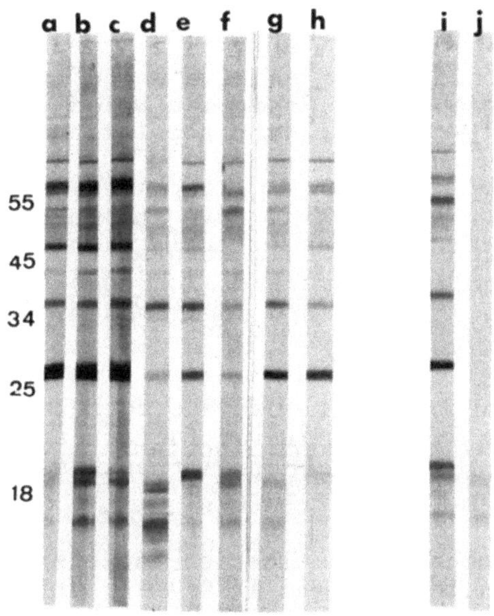

FIGURE 1

Legend of Figure 1: Analysis of sera for antibodies to LAV by Western Blot.

Samples from human sera were tested by the Western blot technique, previously described by Towbin et al. (15).

lanes a, b, f, h	:	sera from AIDS patients
lanes c, d, g	:	sera from patients with AIDS related complexe
lane e	:	serum from an hemophiliac, asymptomatic carrier
lane i	:	positive control serum
lane j	:	negative control serum

Recently, a major glycoprotein has been identified using ^{35}S cysteine labelled virus and immunoprecipitation by patients sera (16). It is a high molecular weight protein (110 K) which is glycosylated. Antibodies to LAV gp110 are detected in almost all patients sera.

4) LAV genome

LAV genome has been recently cloned (17). The size of this genome is 9,1 kb long. No molecular evidence of a relationship between LAV and other human retroviruses (HTLV I and HTLV II) has been found. The complete nucleotide sequence of LAV has been very recently determined by S. Wain-Hobson and coll.(18). They have shown a peculiar genetic structure of LAV with two novel open reading frames, named Q and F, in addition to the conventional retroviral gag-pol-env genes, confirming that LAV may belong to a new group of retroviruses.

III. Evidence for a causal role of LAV in AIDS or ARC

The etiological role of LAV in AIDS and related symptomes is supported by most of the data already mentionned :

1) its frequent isolation from all groups of patients with AIDS or at risk of AIDS

2) its cytopathic effect and its selective tropism for the helper/inducer T lymphocytes, the population of T cells which is mainly affected in the disease.

Moreover, serological data have indicated a high prevalence of antibodies to the virus in patients with AIDS or with ARC as well as in healthy individuals at risk for the disease (4) (19)(20)(21). Table 2 summarizes such results which have been obtained using an ELISA and confirmed by other technics (RIPA or Western blot analysis).

In the group of hemophiliacs, the correlation between the way of treatment by antihemophiliac factors and the percentage of LAV antibodies clearly suggests a transmission of the virus or viral antigens by blood products.

A high percentage of antibodies has also been detected in IV drug abusers in the USA and in France. This confirms also the possible viral transmission via blood or blood products

TABLE II

GROUP	PREVALENCE OF ANTIBODY TO LAV (% positive)
* AIDS patients:	
- Caucasian	75
- Zairian	90
* ARC patients	90
* Risk groups:	
- Healthy homosexuals	20
- Sexual contact of AIDS	50
- Hemophiliacs:	
* heavily treated	60
* lightly treated	10
* General heterosexual population:	
- in France	0,3
- in Zaire	7

which was already suggested by the isolation of the virus from a blood donor recipient pair (22) and from hemophiliac patients (5).

All these data are consistent with the involvment of LAV related viruses in AIDS and its prodromes.

IV. Chemical and physical inactivation of LAV

Since no vaccine is yet available, inactivation of LAV in blood and blood products had to be considered as priority.

Our study on the effect of several commonly used chemical disinfectants on LAV (23) showed that 25 % ethanol solution as well as 1 % glutaraldehyde should be effective for disinfecting medical instruments and that 0,2 % sodium hypochloride inactivated the virus in the first 5 minutes. The reverse transcriptase of LAV is also sensitive to 0,1 % formalin and 1/4000 β propionolactone treatment.

Recently, we described also the effects of physical agents on LAV (24). We demonstrated that LAV is easily inactivated by a 56°C heating during 30 minutes while gamma irradiation with less than 2,5 x 10^5 rads and UV radiations at doses lower than 5 x 10^3 J/m^2 are not sufficient to suppress the infectivity of LAV.

From all these data, useful informations can be drawn for the safety of physicians and laboratory workers.

V. Comparison of LAV and HTLV III viral proteins

Previous reports on the biological and biochemical properties of LAV (2)(3)(4)(10) and HTLV III (7)(8) (25)(26) suggested that both viruses are very similar if not identical.

Comparative studies on their viral proteins have been performed (27). Competitive radioimmunoassays and comparative Western blot analysis indicated the immunological identity between LAV and HTLV III antigens. These data were confirmed by recent reports on nucleotide sequence analysis of both viruses (18)(28).

Thus, as expected, LAV and HTLV III are independent isolates of the same virus.

CONCLUSION

In this paper, we summarized all the evidences indicating that LAV/HTLV III is the causative agent of AIDS. Although the pathogenic role of this new retrovirus is not well known, we have emphasized that repeated LAV/HTLV III infections or repeated antigenic stimuli (bacterial, fungal or viral infections) may contribue to the spreading of the virus since only activated lymphocytes can express the virus (2)(4). The consequence of such viral spread would be first, the lymphadenopathy syndrome in some patients, then the irreversible and severe immune deficiency. This model would also explain why LAV/HTLV III primary infection can lead to an unapparent disease, as it is the case in asymptomatic carriers. But further investigations are required to verify such hypothesis.

However, the discovery of the primary agent of AIDS open the way to the prevention and the treatment of the disease. The prevention of the disease will result from the development of diagnosis methods as well as from the use of viral inactivation methods. Such methods will allow to decrease the transmission of the virus by blood or blood products. For the treatment, one of the possible strategy is to reduce the viral spread using specific inhibitors of the viral reverse transcriptase. Such therapeutic investigations are already in progress (29).

ACKNOWLEDGMENTS

We thank F. Rey, M.T. Nugeyre, S. Chamaret, J. Gruest and D. Guetard for their excellent technical assistance. This work was done in collaboration with L. Montagnier, B.Spire, D. Dormont, D. Klatzmann, J.C. Gluckman, F. Brun, C. Rouzioux, M. Alizon and S. Wain-Hobson. We acknowledge H. Sinno for typing the manuscript. This work was supported by Pasteur Institute, the CNRS and the French National League against Cancer.

REFERENCES

1. F. BARRE-SINOUSSI, J.C. CHERMANN, F.REY et al., Isolation of a T-lymphotropic retrovirus from a patient at risk of acquired immunodeficiency syndrome. Science, 220:868 (1983).

2. J.C.CHERMANN, F. BARRE-SINOUSSI and L. MONTAGNIER. Characterisation and possible role in AIDS of a new human T-lymphotropic retrovirus. In: Acquired immune deficiency syndrome. UCLA Symposia on molecular and cellular biology. New series, Volume 16, Eds. M.S. Gottlieb and J.E. Groopman, Alan R. Liss, Inc., New York, N.Y. 31, (1984).

3. F.BARRE-SINOUSSI, J.C. CHERMANN and L. MONTAGNIER. A new human retrovirus associated with acquired immunodeficiency syndrome (AIDS) or AIDS-related symptoms. In: Manipulation of host defense mechanisms". Ed. Tadao Aoki(JAPAN), 1 vol. (1984), in press.

4. L. MONTAGNIER, J.C. CHERMANN, F. BARRE-SINOUSSI et al., A new human T-lymphotropic retrovirus: characterisation and possible role in lymphadenopathy and acquired immune deficiency syndromes. Cold Spring Harbor publication - Meeting on "Human T-cell leukemia viruses", 1 vol., 363, (1984)

5. E. VILMER, F. BARRE-SINOUSSI, C. ROUZIOUX et al. Isolation of new lymphotropic retrovirus from two siblings with hemophilia B, one with AIDS.
Lancet,i, 753, (1984).

6. A. ELLRODT, F. BARRE-SINOUSSI, P. LE BRAS et al. Isolation of a new human T-lymphotropic retrovirus (LAV) from a marired couple of Zairians, one with AIDS, the other with prodromes. Lancet, i, 1383, (1984).

7. R.C. GALLO, S.Z. SALAHUDDIN, M. POPOVIC et al. Frequent detection and isolation of cytopathic retrovirus (HTLV III) from patients with AIDS and at risk for AIDS. Science, 224, 500, (1984).

8. M. POPOVIC, M.G. SARNGADHARAN, E. READ and R.C. GALLO. Detection, isolation, and continuous production of cytopathic retroviruses (HTLV III) from patients with AIDS and pre-AIDS. Science, 224, 497, (1984).

9. J.A. LEVY, A.D. HOFFMAN, S.M. KRAMER et al. Isolation of lymphocytopathic retroviruses from San Francisco patients with AIDS. Science, 225, 840, (1984).

10. D. KLATZMANN, F. BARRE-SINOUSSI, J.C. CHERMANN et al. Selective tropism for the helper/inducer T-lymphocyte subset of a new human retrovirus associated with the acquired immunodeficiency syndrome. Science, 225, 59, (1984).

11. D. KLATZMANN, E. CHAMPAGNE, S. CHAMARET et al. T-lymphocyte T4 molecule behaves as the receptor for human retrovirus LAV. Nature, 312, 767, (1984).

12. A.G. DALGLEISH, P.C.L. BEVERLEY, P.R. CLAPHAM et al. The CDA (T4) antigen is an essential component of the receptor for the AIDS retrovirus. Nature, 312, 763, (1984).

13. L. MONTAGNIER, C. DAUGUET, C. AXLER et al. A new type of retrovirus isolated from patients presenting with lymphadenopathy and acquired immune deficiency syndrome: Structural and antigenic relatedness with equine infectious anemia virus. Ann. Virol. (Institut Pasteur), 135 E, 119, (1984).

14. F. BARRE-SINOUSSI, J.C. CHERMANN and L. MONTAGNIER. Analysis and Immunological properties of lymphadenopathy associated virus (LAV) structural proteins. Intern. symposium on retroviruses and human pathology, Lerici (Italy), Sept. 1984, Humana Press Inc., (in press).

15. H. TOWBIN, T. STAEHLIN, J. GORDON. Electrophoretic transfer of proteins from polyacrylamide gels to nitrocellulose sheets: procedure and some applications. Proc. Natl. Acad. Sci. U.S.A., 76, 4350, (1979).

16. L. MONTAGNIER, B. KRUST, S.CHAMARET et al. Identification and antigenicity of the major envelope protein of lymphadenopathy associated virus (LAV). J. Virol., (1985), in press.

17. M. ALIZON, P. SONIGO, F. BARRE-SINOUSSI et al. Molecular cloning of lymphadenopathy associated virus. Nature, 312, 757, (1984).

18. S. WAIN-HOBSON, P. SONIGO, O. DANOS et al. Nucleotide sequence of the AIDS virus, LAV. Cell, 40, 9, (1985).

19. F.BRUN-VEZINET, C. ROUZIOUX, F. BARRE-SINOUSSI et al. Detection of IgG antibodies to lymphadenopathy associated virus (LAV) by ELISA, in patients with acquired immunodeficiency syndrome or lymphadenopathy syndrome.Lancet,i,1253, (1984).

20. F. BRUN-VEZINET, C. ROUZIOUX, L. MONTAGNIER et al. Prevalence of antibodies to lymphadenopathy associated retrovirus in African patients with acquired immune deficiency syndrome. Science, 226, 453, (1984).

21. E. MELBYE, R.J. BIGGAR, J.C. CHERMANN et al. High prevalence of lymphadenopathy virus (LAV) in European hemophiliacs. Lancet, ii, 40, (1984).

22. M.P. FEORINO, V.S. KALYANARAMAN, H.W. HAVERKOS et al. Lymphadenopathy Associated Virus (LAV) infection of a blood donor-recipient pair with acquired immunodeficiency syndrome. Science, 225, 69, (1984).

23. B. SPIRE, F. BARRE-SINOUSSI, L. MONTAGNIER and J.C. CHERMANN Inactivation of Lymphadenopathy Associated Virus by chemical disinfectants. Lancet, ii, 899, (1984).

24. B. SPIRE, D. DORMONT, F. BARRE-SINOUSSI et al. Inactivation of Lymphadenopathy Associated Virus by heat, gamma rays, and ultraviolet light. Lancet, i, 188, (1985).

25. M.G. SARNGADHARAN, M. POPOVIC, L. BRUCH et al. Antibodies reactive with human T-lymphotropic retroviruses (HTLV III) in the serum of patients with AIDS. Science, 224, 506, (1984).

26. J. SCHUPBACH, M. POPOVIC, R.V. GILDEN et al. Serological analysis of a subgroup of human T-lymphotropic retroviruses (HTLV III) associated with AIDS. Science, 224, 503, (1984).

27. J.C. CHERMANN, M.S. SARNGADHARAN, F. BARRE-SINOUSSI et al. (in preparation).

28. L. RATNER, W. HASELTINE, R. PATARCA et al. Complete nucleotide sequence of the AIDS virus, HTLV III. Nature, vol.313, 600, 277, (1985).

29. W. ROZENBAUM, D. DORMONT, B. SPIRE et al. Antimoniotungstate (HPA 23) treatment of 4 patients with AIDS or prodromes. Lancet, i,(1985), in press.

EXPRESSIONS OF HTLV-III INFECTION IN A PEDIATRIC POPULATION

Savita Pahwa, Senih Fikrig, Mark Kaplan, Ellen Kahn, and Rajendra Pahwa

North Shore University Hospital, Manhasset, New York, Cornell University Medical College & Downstate Medical Center Brooklyn, New York, State University of New York

INTRODUCTION

The etiologic agent for the acquired immunodeficiency syndrome (AIDS) has now been identified as being a lymphocytotropic retrovirus, designated as HTLV-III (human T-cell lymphocytotropic virus III) and the LAV/IDAV (lymphadenopathy associated virus/ immunodeficiency associated virus).[1-3] It is now clear that the disease can occur in children as well,[4-7] characteristically inflicting offspring of women in risk groups and recipients of blood transfusions and blood products. Prior to knowledge of the etiologic agent for AIDS, the Centers for Disease Control (CDC) developed a working definition of AIDS for purposes of national surveillance, which was extended for children as well.[4] This definition served a very useful purpose, but its strict inclusionary criteria resulted in exclusion of many cases which, after going through a series of terminologies, subsequently got collectively termed as AIDS-related complex or ARC. Conforming to these definitions has been especially problematic in children who have certain unique features not seen in adults. It is the purpose of this report to discuss characteristic features in a group of pediatric patients from Long Island and Brooklyn in metropolitan New York. We have considered evidence for HTLV III infection as the single requisite for inclusion in the study, and here we discuss the spectrum of clinical and laboratory manifestations that may be associated with HTLV III infection in children.

METHODS

Peripheral Blood Studies

Serologic testing for HTLV III antibody was performed by Western blot analysis.[8] Specifically, presence of antibody to the p41 antigen was considered evidence of seropositivity. T cell subsets were quantitated in whole blood by flow cytometry, using Ortho Spectrum III and Orthoclone monoclonal antibodies, OKT3, OKT4, OKT8 and OKT11 (Ortho Diagnostic Division, New Jersey). Proliferative responses of peripheral blood lymphocytes to mitogens phytohemagglutinin (PHA), concanavalin A (Con A), and pokeweed mitogen (PWM), was tested by C^{14} thymidine incorporation. Quantitative serum immunoglobulins were determined by nephelometry, and levels of serum thymic hormone, thymulin were determined as previously described.[9]

Tissue Studies

Biopsy material from liver was available in three patients and from lung in two. The tissue was subjected to routine culturing for bacteria and fungus, and special culturing for cytomegalovirus (CMV). Examination for protozoa, i.e. pneumocystis carinii, was also done. A portion of each biopsy was snap frozen in a dry ice-acetone bath and stored at -60 degrees Centigrade for lymphocyte subset determination. The method of staining with monoclonal antibodies was a modification of the Avidin-Biotin-Peroxidase Complex (ABC) technique described by Hsu et al.[10] Staining was performed with monoclonal antibodies, Leu 2a, 3a, 4 (Becton-Dickinson), and B1 (Coulter). Color reaction was produced with 3-amino-9-ethyl carbazole (Sigma), and sections were counterstained with Mayer's hematoxylin (Sigma). In the liver, lymphocytes in portal spaces and lobules were counted and areas of lymphoid nodules were counted in the lung. For light microscopy, formalin-fixed, paraffin-embedded tissue was stained with hematoxylin-eosin. Periodic acid-Schiff (PAS) with and without diastase digestion, reticulin, trichrome, elastic van Gieson, acid-fast bacilli, and Gomori methenamine silver stains were also performed.

RESULTS

Patients: Clinical and Immunologic Characteristics

We have grouped all patients with clinical evidence of disease and positive serology for HTLV III into Group I. In this group, we have categorized patients based on clinical characteristics (Table 1). Of the 15 patients in this group, 6 who had opportunistic infections and thus qualified for the CDC definition of pediatric AIDS were placed in category 1a. Because of the high incidence of serious bacterial infections in children as opposed to adults with AIDS, we have included serious bacterial infection in the same category as opportunistic infection (Category 1a). Of importance is to note occurrence of lymphocytic interstitial pneumonitis (Category 1b) and salivary gland enlargement (Category 1c) in some pediatric patients. Also notable is the occurrence of central nervous system manifestations including congenital malformations in this patient population (Category 1d). One patient had disseminated immunoblastic lymphoma and was categorized under malignancies (1e). All patients in Group I had at least one "common characteristic" listed under category 1e. Immune abnormalities were present in all patients from Group I. Patients with none or minimal significant clinical manifestations are grouped into Groups IIA (1 patient) and IIB (2 patients). They were distinguished on the basis of immunologic abnormalities which were present only in Group IIA. Immunologic abnormalities most frequently noted in patients from Groups I and II are listed in Table 2.

Liver Histopathology

Lobular and portal changes of varying degrees were noted, and consisted of hyperplasia of the sinusoidal lining cells and lymphocytic infiltration in a diffuse or nodular distribution in lobules and in portal spaces associated with piecemeal necrosis. Bile duct damage and moderate portal fibrosis were noted. Special stains, specifically AFB, revealed no micro-organisms. No nuclear inclusions were found in the specimens.

Lung Histopathology

The lung pattern was that of an interstitial pneumonia characterized by widening of the interalveolar septae by a diffuse lymphoplasmacytic infiltrate. These changes were associated with narrowing of the corresponding air spaces, and alveolar cell hyperplasia. Nodular mononuclear infiltrates were also present, at times related to the bronchioli in an eccentric or concentric fashion. Granuloma and nuclear inclusions were not found, and all special stains were negative.

TABLE 1

CLINICAL CATEGORIES OF GROUP I DISEASE IN 15 CHILDREN

(Inclusive of AIDS and ARC)

Categories	Clinical Characteristics	# Positive
1a	Serious Infections	
	-Opportunistic infections alone	4
	-Severe bacterial infections alone (pneumonia, meningitis, sepsis)	4
	-Opportunistic infection plus severe bacterial infection	2
1b	Lymphocytic interstitial pneumonitis	6
1c	Salivary gland enlargement	2
1d	Central nervous system involvement (brain atrophy, microcephaly, "encephalopathies")	3
1e	Malignancies: immunoblastic lymphoma	1
1f	Common characteristics	
	-lymphadenopathy (2 or more sites)	15
	-hepatomegaly/splenomegaly	12/6
	-diarrhea	3
	-upper respiratory tract infections and otitis media	10
	-thrush and candidal skin infections	11
	-failure to thrive	10

Tissue Lymphocyte Phenotyping

There was a predominance of T cells in all lymphocytic infiltrates of liver and lung. T8 cells accounted for the majority of T cells with quantitatively fewer T4 lymphocytes. Only a sparse scattering of B cells were noted in the tissues.

TABLE 2

IMMUNE ABNORMALITIES IN PEDIATRIC HTLV III INFECTIONS

GROUPS I AND IIA

	No. Abn.	No. Tested	% Abn.
Hypergammaglobulinemia (IgG ± others)	16	16	100
Lymphopenia of T4 cells with reversal of T4/T8 ratio (< 1.0)	14	16	87
Depressed responses to one or more mitogens	9	12	75
Reduced thymulin levels	12	12	100

DISCUSSION

In this report we focus attention on pediatric AIDS, as being only part of a broad spectrum of diseases resulting from infection with HTLV III. Serologic studies performed in large numbers of patients with AIDS and ARC as well as in individuals in risk and non-risk groups have shown rather definitively that presence of antibody to HTLV III is indicative of infection with the virus in most risk groups[8] with the possible exception of hemophiliacs. Individuals in non-risk groups have remained consistently seronegative. Now that the etiologic agent for AIDS has been established and individuals exposed to the virus can be identified, we feel that a re-evaluation of diseases associated with HTLV III infection is in order, with special emphasis on the various manifestations of what is currently termed ARC.

In this report we have offered an alternative approach (not necessarily the best one) for classifying AIDS and ARC like disorders in children taking seropositivity for HTLV III as the criterion for inclusion. So as not to minimize the importance of certain clinical characteristics and thereby hinder recognition of this disease we have included all patients with significant clinical manifestations into one group, (Group I). However, in an attempt not to completely diverge from previous terminology, all patients with severe opportunistic infections (i.e. those qualifying for the CDC diagnosis of AIDS) have been placed into a separate category, la, in which we have also included patients with serious bacterial infections, as such infections pose a real threat for this population. We have brought to attention once again features previously recognized[5-7] as being unique to the pediatric population viz lymphocytic interstitial pneumonitis and salivary gland enlargement. Additionally, we would like to emphasize the occurrence of significant central nervous system disease, which may present at the time of birth as congenital malformation i.e. brain atrophy and microcephaly or present later as an encephalopathy as comprising part of the clinical spectrum of HTLV III infection in children.

Investigation of histopathology of liver in patients with Group I disease who had hepatomegaly revealed a chronic active hepatitis-like picture. This pathology was associated with elevated serum transaminases.[11] Lung tissue in patients with interstitial pneumonitis revealed lymphocytic infiltrates similiar to those described before by others.[12] In both tissues the T8 subset of lymphocytes predominated. This phenomenon of lymphocytic infiltration in tissues presumably reflects an immunologic reaction to an agent, most likely viral in nature. As cultures in tissues were negative for cytomegalovirus and inclusion bodies were not seen, the most probable candidates are HTLV III and Epstein Barr virus (EBV). Immunologic reaction in peripheral blood following EBV infection is one of suppressor/cytotoxic (T8) cell proliferation[13] as a means of curbing the infectious agent. A similar mechanism of immune activation might be operational in tissues of HTLV III infected pediatric patients in response to the HTLV III virus alone or in association with a cofactor such as EBV, infection with EBV being almost universal in patients with AIDS.

Our observations indicate that laboratory abnormalities are almost always present in individuals with HTLV III infection, even in asymptomatic children. The single exception in our present population was an asymptomatic child of a mother with AIDS. This child, although seropositive, did not have demonstrable laboratory abnormalities. The most frequently noted laboratory abnormalities were hypergammaglobulinemia, marked imbalance in T cell subsets with T4 lymphopenia and decreased serum thymulin levels. Such a triad is unusual in most other clinical entities including primary immunodeficiency diseases, and should serve to alert physicians to the possibility of HTLV III infection, especially in children that fall into "at risk" categories. A number of other immunologic abnormalities have been reported in patients with AIDS or ARC, including elevated β2 microglobulin[14] increased acid labile interferon[15], decreased lymphokine production[16] and abnormal B cell proliferation and differentiation responses[17,18]. Systematic evaluation of these parameters has not been made as yet in children with AIDS or ARC. B cell dysfunction in-vitro similar to that observed in adults has however been noted in children, (Pahwa, S. unpublished observation). Clinically, functional B cell deficiency is of great significance in the pediatric population because the latter, unlike adults are extremely prone to recurrent bacterial infections. The functional B cell impairment also provides a rationale for intravenous gammaglobulin therapy in pediatric AIDS[19]. The almost universal presence of thymic epithelial injury, as evidenced by decreased thymic hormone secretory capacity, is also highly significant when considered in the context of developing therapeutic strategies.

The heterogeneity in clinical expression of HTLV III infection was brought sharply into focus by the identification of three seropositive children without clinical manifestations whom we placed in groups IIA & IIB distinguishable by presence or absence of immunolgic abnormalities listed in Table II. Recognition of infected but asymptomatic individuals is specially important for understanding the biologic variations in HTLV III infections from the point of view of the host and the agent, for recognition of carrier states and in understanding modes of transmission of this infectious agent. The latter point is particularly relevant for adults who might serve as potential blood donors. Our selection criteria have excluded another population, who might be virus positive but seronegative. Evidence for such states is already documented[20]. Table 3 depicts our concept of possible general groups of children (or adults) with HTLV III infection.

TABLE 3

CLASSIFICATION OF INDIVIDUALS INFECTED WITH HTLV III VIRUS

Group	Antibody	Clinical Abnormalities	Immunologic Abnormalities A/B
I	+	+	+/-
II	+	—	+/-
III	—	+	+/-
IV	—	—	+/-

With respect to childhood infections with HTLV III, Groups III and IV might be especially relevant in the very young infant because of innate immaturity of B cells in the newborn period. Ideally therefore, virus isolation coupled with serology would be most informative in investigations of the disease. Within each group, one would expect further categorization based on clinical abnormalities, as we have observed for Group I. At the present time it is not clear which category other than la in Group I carries a worse prognosis, and to what extent there is overlap between the various categories.

In conclusion, we believe that overt manifestations of HTLV III infection in children comprise a disease entity distinct from hitherto described disorders of primary and secondary immunodeficiency diseases. We are just beginning to appreciate that what we have been recognizing thus far represents but the tip of an iceberg. Many questions remain and many issues need to be addressed in depth. Among the latter, one of primary importance is the mode of acquisition of infection in children. While most reported data implicates vertical spread in-utero from mother to child, this issue clearly needs further investigation to rule out perinatal and horizontal spread of infection. An awareness of subtle expressions of virus-host interaction should lead to indepth exploration and understanding of the manifaceted spectrum associated with infection with HTLV III.

ACKNOWLEDGEMENT

We are grateful to Dr. M.G. Sarngadharan of Litton Bionetics Inc. for performing viral serology, to Dr. G. Incefy for performing serum thymulin assays, to Dr. L. Duffy for phenotypic analysis of lymphocytes in liver biopsies, to Corinne Leombruno and Maria Marecki for technical assistance and to Ann Abbatiello for secretarial assistance.

REFERENCES

1. R. C. Gallo,P. S. Sarin, and E. P. Gelmann, et al,Isolation of human T cell leukemia virus in acquired immune deficiency syndrome (AIDS), Sci. 220:865-867 (1983).
2. S. Border, R. C. Gallo, A pathogenic retrovirus (HTLV III) linked to AIDS, N. Engl. J. Med. 511:1292-1297 (1984).
3. M. Seligman, L. Chess, J. L. Fahey, A. S. Fauci, P. J. Lachmann, J. L'Age-stehr, J. Ngu, A. J. Panching, F. S. Rosen, T. J. Spira and J. Wybran, AIDS - An immunologic reevaluation, N. Eng. J. Med. 311:1286-1292 (1984).
4. P. A. Thomas, H. W. Jaffe, T. J. Spira, R. Reiss, I. C. Guerrero, and D. Auerbach, Unexplained immunodeficiency in children, J. Am. Med. Assoc. 252:639-644 (1984).
5. J. Oleska, A. Minnefor, R. Cooper, K. Thomas, A. Dela Cruz, H. Ahdieh, I. Guerrero, V. V. Joshi, and F. Desposito, Immune deficiency syndrome in children, J. Am. Med. Assoc. 249:2345-2349 (1983).
6. G. B. Scott, B. E. Buck, J. G. Leterman, F. L. Bloom and N. P. Parks, Acquired immunodeficiency syndrome in infants, N. Engl. J. Med. 310:76-81 (1984).
7. A. Rubinstein, Acquired immunodeficiency syndrome in infants, Am. J. Dis. Child. 137:825-827 (1983).
8. M. G. Sarngadharan, M. Popovic, J. Schupback, and R. C. Gallo, Antibodies reactive with human T-lymphotropic retrovirus (HTLV III) in the serum of patients with AIDS. Sci 224:506-508.

9. T. Iwata, G. S. Incefy, S. Cunningham-Rundles, C. Cunningham-Rundles, E. Smithwick, N. Geller, R. O'Reilly, and R. A. Good, Circulating thymic hormones in patients with primary and secondary immune deficiency disease, Am. J. Med. 71:385-394 (1981).
10. S. Hsu, L. Raine, H. Fanger, Use of Avidin-Biotin-Peroxidase Complex (ABC) in immunoperoxidase techniques: A comparison between ABC and unlabeled antibody (PAP) procedures, J. of Histochem. and Cytochem. 29(4):577-580 (1981).
11. L. Duffy, S. Pahwa, E. Kahn, S. Teichberg, J. Fagin, K. Kenigsberg, S. E. Fisher, and F. Daum, Hepatitis in children with AIDS, Histopathologic and immunocytologic features. Submitted for publication.
12. V. V. Joshi, J. M. Oleske, A. B. Minnefor, S. Saad, K. M. Klein, R. Sign, M. Zabala, C. Dadzie, M. Simpser, R. H. Rapkin, Pulmonary pathology of acquired immunodeficiency syndrome (AIDS) in children. A study of ten cases. Human Pathology. In Press.
13. E. L. Reinherz, C. O'Brien, P. Rosenthal, S. F. Schlossman, The cellular basis for viral induced immunodeficiency: analysis by monoclonal antibodies, J. Immunol. 125:1269 (1980).
14. S. Zolla-Pazner, D. William, W. El-Sadr, M. Marmor, and R. Stahl, Quantitation of B_2-microglobulin and other immune characteristics in a prospective study of men at risk for acquired immunodeficiency syndrome, J. Am. Med. Assoc. 251:2951-2955 (1984).
15. E. DeStafano, R. M. Friedman, A. E. Friedman-Kien, et al, Acid labile human leukocyte interferon in homosexual men with kaposi's sarcoma and lymphadenopathy, J. Inf. Dis. 146:451-415 (1982).
16. N. Talal, G. Shearer, A clinician and a scientist look at acquired immunodeficiency syndrome, Immunol. Today 4:180-185 (1983).
17. C. H. Lane, H. Masur, and L. C. Edgar, et al, Abnormalities of B-cell activation and immunoregulation in patients with the acquired immunodeficiency syndrome, N. Engl. J. Med. 309:453-458 (1983).
18. S. G. Pahwa, M. T. J. Quilop, M. Lange, R. N. Pahwa, and M. H. Grieco, Defective B lymphocyte function in homosexual men in relation to the acquired immunodeficiency syndrome. Ann. Int. Med. In Press.
19. J. E. Groopman, S. Z. Salahuddin, M. G. Sarnadharan, et al, Virologic studies in a case of transfusion-associated AIDS, N. Eng. J. Med. 311:1419-1422 (1984).
20. A. Rubinstein, M. Sicklick, L. Bernstein, B. Silverman, B. Novick, M. Charytan and B. Krieger, Treatment of AIDS with intravenous gammaglobulin, Ped. Res. 18:264A (1984).

ROLE OF EPSTEIN-BARR VIRUS IN ACQUIRED IMMUNE DEFICIENCY SYNDROME

David T. Purtilo[1,2,3], Helen Kipscomb[1,3], Gerhard Krueger[4], Joseph Sonnabend[5], Dominic Casareale[1], and David J. Volsky[1,3]

[1]Department of Pathology and Laboratory Medicine,
[2]Pediatrics, The University of Nebraska Medical Center
[3]The Eppley Institute for Research in Cancer and Allied Diseases, 42nd and Dewey Avenue, Omaha, Nebraska 68105
[4]Immunopathology Laboratories, Pathology Institute University of Cologne, Clinical Center Lindenburg 5000 Cologne 41, West Germany
[5]49 West 12 Street, New York, New York 10011

INTRODUCTION

Human lymphotropic viruses including human T cell leukemia virus-III (HTLV-III), Epstein-Barr virus (EBV), and cytomegalovirus (CMV) likely serve important etiological roles in the induction of the acquired immune deficiency syndrome (AIDS) and in the AIDS-related malignancies. By infecting the cellular components of the immune system, these viruses alter the balance between the various lymphocyte subpopulations and affect immune regulation as well.[1-3] HTLV-III is thought to be important in the induction of AIDS, especially for the final stages in the pathogenesis, owing to infection and lysis of T helper cells. CMV and EBV have been implicated in the induction of both benign and malignant disorders in patients with AIDS, including Kaposi's sarcoma and malignant B cell lymphoma, respectively.[4]

Following a brief introduction regarding the biological characteristics of EBV and the immune effector mechanisms normally controlling this ubiquitous virus, we will summarize a spectrum of diseases that occur in immune deficient patients. Individuals who have developed AIDS including hemophiliacs, Haitians, intravenous heroin users, young children born of mothers using intravenous heroin, and male homosexuals will be discussed regarding the role of EBV in the pathogenesis of their diseases. Since 1982 we have studied and compared male homosexuals from Greenwich Village and Omaha. We will compare and contrast the findings in these two populations regarding EBV serology and comment on hematopathological aspects of patients studied in Cologne in West Germany. Our discussion will conclude with a hypothesis concerning interactions between EBV and HTLV-III in the induction of AIDS.

Biological Characteristics of EBV

EBV is a ubiquitous human Herpesvirus. Other members of this group include CMV, varicella-zoster, and herpes simplex. EBV predominantly infects human B lymphocytes, owing to the presence of specific viral receptors on B cells.[2] The infection usually results in B cell transformation rather than virus replication. Lytic or productive infection most likely occurs in the epithelial cells of oropharynx or parotid ductular cells.[5,6,7] During acute infection, most individuals shed virus in their saliva whereas during latency only a minority of patients shed virus. The immune response to EBV seems to be the major determinant of the outcome of infections.[8]

Immunologic Surveillance against EBV

Initial barriers to EBV infection include the lack of viral receptors on most cells (other than B cells), natural killing (NK) of virally infected cells, and the anti-viral impact of interferon.[9] The vast majority of individuals become asymptomatically infected with EBV during childhood.[5] In contrast, approximately 50-65% of adolescents or young adults develop self-limiting infectious mononucleosis (IM) on primary infection.

EBV evokes a potent response from the immune system in individuals who develop IM: a polyclonal proliferation of B cells and activation of cytotoxic T cells (CTL) and macrophages is observed. Hence, the patients develop lymphocytosis, lymphadenomegaly, and splenomegaly.[10] Monoclonal antibody marking of the cells reveals that the majority of the cells are suppressor-lytic T lymphocytes.[11] Only about 2% of the circulating B cells possess EBV genome, however, depletion of T cells from peripheral blood and then culturing B cells for 18-24 hours results in 6-20% EBV genome positivity of B cells.[12]

Infection of B lymphocytes by EBV in-vitro results in a polyclonal B cell activation and immunoglobulin synthesis.[13] In-vivo, this is manifested by significantly increased serum levels of IgM, IgG, and IgA. A minority of the immunoglobulin synthesis is directed towards EBV specific antigens, including viral capsid antigen (VCA), early antigen (EA), and EB nuclear-associated antigen (EBNA). Heterophile antibodies are produced as part of the polyclonal burst of immunoglobulin synthesis. Problematic to the patient is the development of autoantibodies including those against neutrophils,[14] platelets, and erythrocytes (reviewed in 15). Rheumatoid factor and anti-nuclear antibodies may also form. An array of diseases can result from EBV infection. The clinical results of infection by the virus depend on whether the individual has an immune deficiency and the type, degree of deficiency, and timing of the infection with respect to onset of immune deficiency.

Spectrum of EBV-induced Diseases: XLP Model

The X-linked lymphoproliferative syndrome (XLP) is a model for studying EBV-induced diseases in immune deficient patients.[16] Owing to inheritance of a defective lymphoproliferative control locus on the X chromosome, EBV evokes aproliferative diseases including red cell aplasia, aplastic anemia, hypogammaglobulinemia and proliferative diseases including fatal or chronic infectious mononucleosis (IM), pseudolymphoma or malignant B cell lymphoma in males with XLP.[17] The IM phenotype is manifested by polyclonal elevation of serum Ig, lymphadenomegaly and splenomegaly. Necrosis of vital organs, especially the liver, is associated with lymphocytic infiltration.[18] Uncontrolled NK and cytotoxic T cells may be responsible for destruction of these organs.

Survivors tend to show hypogammaglobulinemia or malignant lymphoma phenotypes. They also show an increased number of suppressor T cells and diminished helper T cell populations. Despite their multiple immune defects including NK, CTL, antibody, and memory T cells,[19] some patients are able to survive. This survival of about 15% of the patients may be due to retention of defense against EBV by antibody-dependent cellular cytotoxicity.[20]

Patients with inherited immune deficiency disorders such as ataxia-telangiectasia and Wiskott-Aldrich syndrome and those with acquired immune deficiency syndromes such as renal transplant recipients and AIDS can also experience EBV-induced lymphoproliferative diseases.[8] It seems reasonable that patients with AIDS would also develop a spectrum of EBV-associated diseases. In the next section we will address the possible role of EBV in AIDS and the association of the virus with various manifestations of pre-AIDS and AIDS.

Epstein-Barr Virus and Patients at Risk for AIDS

Male homosexuals, intravenous heroin users, Haitians, hemophiliacs, and children born of intravenous drug users have been the predominant groups affected by AIDS. Mucosal contact or parenteral introduction of an agent or agents seems to be necessary for the induction of the syndrome.

Rubinstein et al.[21] and Oleske et al.[22] have described an AIDS-like disease with reversed helper/suppressor T cell ratios in infants born of promiscuous and/or drug-addicted mothers. The onset of the syndrome begins from the neonatal period to nine months of age. The patients show failure to thrive, fever, thrush, Pneumocystis carinii pneumonia, generalized lymphadenomegaly, and hepatosplenomegaly. Their immunologic perturbation is manifested by reversed ratios of T cells, hyperimmunoglobulinemia, and cellular immune defects. Rubinstein et al.[21] have shown that these patients exhibit high titer anti-VCA and EA antibody responses. They have postulated that EBV plays a significant role in the induction of this disorder. We think that other viruses, microbial agents, and the immunosuppressive impact of opiates[23] may also impair immune responses of the children.[4]

Hemophiliacs were noted in the late 1970's to show immune perturbation as evidenced by splenomegaly (Peter Levine-personal communication). At greatest risk were individuals receiving Factor VIII concentrates. These concentrates were prepared from 1975 onward by pooling Factor VIII from 2,000 to 25,000 donors per lot of concentrate. Since an average patient receives three injections per month, the immune system is exposed to multiple antigens. Curiously, the hemophiliac patients who have developed AIDS have almost invariably shown Pneumocystis carinii infection and not Kaposi's sarcoma. Rarely Burkitt's lymphoma has occurred. EBV reactivation and elevation of anti-EA titers is shown in a minority of the patients, however, findings that VCA titers increase, virus is excreted in the oropharynx, and spontaneous lymphoblastoid transformation of peripheral blood leukocytes suggests that reactivation has occurred.[24] Recently, we have studied a 15-year-old male hemophiliac with lymphadenopathy, reversed helper and suppressor T cell ratios, hepatitis B virus induced hepatitis, and reactivation of EBV. A lymph node biopsy specimen contained EBV genome (unpublished observations).

Intravenous drug abusers have accounted for approximately 20% of cases of AIDS.[25] This has occurred predominantly in men in "shooting galleries" in New York City where individuals exchange dirty syringes. Opiates are known to bind with T cells[23] and depress cellular immunity. Concurrent infections with hepatitis and other agents occur. EBV could become reactivated in such a setting owing to depression of immune surveillance mechanisms.

Initially, Haitians were regarded as being a risk group for AIDS.[26,27] The basis for the immune suppression is unknown, however, homosexuality and intravenous drug abuse are common in this group. This recent finding and the possible social stigmatization[28] of a nation may be reasons why Haitians have recently been dropped from the risk group category. An important component of immune deficiency may stem from the low socioeconomic level of Haitians. Poverty is often linked with poor sanitation, undernutrition, parasitism, and immune deficiency. "Nutritional thymectomy" and frequent infections account for concurrent immunostimulation and immunosuppression in these patients.[29]

AIDS has occurred predominantly in a sub-group of male homosexuals having sexual contact with a large number of partners.[30] Manifestations have included autoimmune disturbances, opportunistic infections, Kaposi's sarcoma, chronic lymphadenomegaly, non-Hodgkin's lymphoma, or squamous cell carcinoma. The hypothesis of a single etiologic agent for AIDS, receiving most consideration, is discussed in detail elsewhere in this volume, especially as related to HTLV-III. An alternative view, of Sonnabend et al.,[30] considers that repeated sexual involvement with multiple partners in a sub-group of male homosexuals, exposes the men to the immunosuppressive impact of CMV, and other microbes, drugs and allogeneic semen. We have proposed a biphasic process consisting initially of a reversible acquisition phase of impaired T cell immunoregulation permitting reactivation of EBV, and antibodies produced by the activated B cells. With time, immune defects including destruction of thymic epithelium lead to a second, self-sustaining phase wherein cytotoxic lymphocytes fail to eliminate herpesvirus. Proliferating virally infected cells could lead to CMV-carrying Kaposi's sarcoma and EBV-carrying B cell lymphomas.

Studies Regarding EBV and AIDS in Male Homosexuals

Briefly summarized here are the results of our studies performed on patients from Greenwich Village and Omaha in the United States and Cologne, West Germany. Our studies of male homosexuals at risk for AIDS which began in 1982 have included approximately 230 men from New York City and 68 from Omaha. The majority of patients were in the third through fifth decades of life. In addition, 54 male homosexuals from Cologne, West Germany were independently studied by one of us (G.K.).[31]

Noteworthy, all but one of the 308 homosexual men that we had studied were EBV-seropositive (Table 1). In contrast, our study of adult male controls revealed seropositivity in 91% of men.[32] This percentage is consistent with Henles' data regarding healthy adults with seropositivity.[5] Others have described an unusually high frequency of infectious mononucleosis occurring years before the onset of the syndrome.[33] Moreover, symptoms consisting of chronic lymphadenomegaly, fatigue and pharyngitis are seen in some men with the pre-AIDS syndrome. These are features of chronic infectious mononucleosis (CIM) or chronic active EBV infection.[34] A CIM study we began in 1980 of 29 patients with persistent low grade malaise, fever, pharyngitis, and lymphadenomegaly revealed that three of the patients were male homosexuals. The patients had been studied a year prior to recognition of AIDS. Among male homosexuals, IgA anti-VCA titers tended to be highest in the lymphadenomegaly group and patients with AIDS. Consistently, anti-EA titers indicating viral reactivity were higher in the male homosexuals than in controls as were most groups for their serum IgM, IgA, IgG levels (Table 2).

Table 1. Epstein-Barr Virus-Specific Antibodies in Male Homosexuals

Group	#	% S.P.	anti-VCA IgM %+	anti-VCA IgM GMT	anti-VCA IgA %+	anti-VCA IgA GMT	anti-VCA IgG %+	anti-VCA IgG GMT	anti-EA D %+	anti-EA D GMT	anti-EA DR %+	anti-EA DR GMT	anti-EBNA %+	anti-EBNA GMT
Heterosexual Men, adult	23	91	0	-	0	-	100	74	0	-	14	8	95	32
Homosexual men from Omaha, NE:														
Healthy	58	98	4	a	11	5	100	61	2	b	16	7	98	48
LAD	4	100	0	-	0	-	100	113	0	-	0	-	100	48
AIDS	6	100	0	-	17	c	100	90	0	-	33	d	100	22
Homosexual men from Greenwich Village, NY														
Healthy	57	100	0	-	9	7	100	93	0	-	21	7	93	41
LAD	126	100	3	5	17	7	100	145	4	61	22	18	98	47
KS	17	100	8	e	18	25	100	111	12	f	18	16	94	48
OI	31	100	0	-	35	12	100	156	3	g	16	9	97	42
KS and OI	9	100	0	-	33	6	100	235	0	-	33	5	100	50

Abbreviations: SP = seropositivity; VCA = viral capsid antigen; EA = early antigen; EBNA = EB nuclear-associated antigen; LAD = lymphadenopathy; AIDS = acquired immune deficiency syndrome; KS = Kaposi's sarcoma; OI = opportunistic infections.

[a] N=2, titers=1:5
[b] N=1, titer=1:5
[c] N=1, titer=80
[d] N=2, titer=1:5, 1:20
[e] N=1, titer=40
[f] N=2, titer=1:10, 1:40
[g] N=1, titer=10

Table 2. Plasma Immunoglobulin Concentration (mg/dl) in Male Homosexuals

	IgM	IgA	IgG
Normal range, adult males	60-250	90-450	800-1800
Homosexual men from Omaha, NE:			
Healthy (N=24)	207±93 *	266±186**	1286±225
LAD (N=4)	191±101	185±53	1739±524
AIDS (N=6)	272±197	491±268	1740±448
Homosexual men from Greenwich Village, NY:			
Healthy (N=56)	185±91	256±121	1437±465
LAD (N=113)	232±171	255±154	1902±679
KS only (N=17)	275±149	507±330	2262±419
OI only (N=30)	248±161	540±272	1872±504
KS and OI (N=8)	168±103	359±198	1857±445

Abbreviations: LAD = lymphadenopathy; AIDS = acquired immune deficiency; KS = Kaposi's sarcoma; OI = opportunistic infections
*= N=24; ** N=24, one value = 1,055

The immune system changes dynamically during stages of development from pre-AIDS to AIDS. Lymph node biopsy specimens from 54 patients from Cologne were studied by one of us (G.K.). Lymph nodes demonstrated progressive changes which correlated fairly well with pre-AIDS and AIDS stages. Enlarged lymph nodes in stage I (lymphadenopathy syndrome) exhibited a striking follicular and diffuse (paracortical) hyperplasia. Proliferating follicles contained numerous nuclear-debris-ladden macrophages indicating enhanced cellular turnover. The hyperplastic paracortex frequently showed diffuse and nodular arrangements of basophilic lymphoblasts resembling to some extent infectious mononucleosis. Increased numbers of plasmacytoid cells expanded the medullary cords and tended to infiltrate the paracortex. Occasional micro-focal necrosis or epithelioid cell granulomas were also seen. Immunohistological staining revealed a balanced T helper and T suppressor cell distribution and a marked B cell hyperplasia (follicular and diffuse). In stage II, follicular hyperplasia of lymph nodes persisted and the lymphoplasmacytoid (B cell) population in medullary cords appeared strikingly increased. Plasma cells focally infiltrated the cortical follicle. The paracortex (T zone) contained reduced numbers of small lymphocytes and became focally atrophic; postcapillary venules were inactive with flat endothelia and sclerotic basal lamella. There was also some stromal fibrosis. Nests of plasma cells and histiocytes were found in the paracortex. Diffuse reactive histiocytosis frequently became very extensive and sometimes necrotizing granulomas were seen. The granulomas apparently depended on the type of superimposed infections (i.e., M. avium-intracellare). Focally, increased prominence of postcapillary venules with suggestive vascular proliferation was seen. In this stage, as in stage III, immunohistological reactions exhibited a striking decrease in T helper cells with a concomitant increase in T suppressor cells and polyclonal B lymphocytes.

In stage III (AIDS) the structure of the enlarged lymph nodes was obliterated by a diffuse lymphoplasmacytic cell proliferation associated with variable amounts of immunoblasts, reticulo-histiocytic cells and more or less obvious angioproliferation. It was difficult or impossible to recognize cortical, paracortical or medullary structures. The lesion resembled to some extent lymphoplasmacytoid lymphoma, angioimmunoblastic lympadenopathy, or even polymorphic immunoblastic lymphoma. However, immunohistological staining demonstrated polyclonal B cell populations and thus reactive lymphoid cellular populations. Additional morphological descriptions of the lymph nodes in male homosexuals can be found in reference 31.

The role of EBV in the induction of the lymphadenomegaly is controversial. Crawford et al.[35] have studied 25 homosexual men, 14 of whom had persistent lymphadenomegaly. All were seropositive and 11 had antibodies to EA. Thirteen of 17 excreted virus in their saliva and two showed defective memory T cell function. Peripheral blood lymphocytes from 6 of the patients failed to reveal EBNA staining by immunofluorescence as did lymph node biopsy specimens from 5 patients. In contrast, we have found EBV genome in 4 of 6 lymph nodes studied by molecular hybridization (unpublished observations).[32] Noteworthy, two of our four patients containing EBV genome in their lymph nodes did not serologically show reactivation of virus. Molecular hybridization is likely a more sensitive technique than staining for EBNA by immunofluorescence in touch imprints of lymph nodes. Data regarding the role of EBV in the induction of the malignant B cell neoplasms in the patients also substantially establishes a relationship of the virus and their lymphadenomegaly.

Since 1981, 90 malignant lymphomas (almost all non-Hodgkin's lymphomas) have occurred where AIDS is seen in Los Angeles, New York, and San Francisco hospitals.[36] Hodgkin's disease is uncommonly seen in patients with primary and secondary immunodeficiency disorders. This is likely due to the vulnerability to EBV of immune deficient patients and thus the resultant B cell lymphomas.[8] In contrast, Hodgkin's disease tissues do not contain EBV. Zeigler et al.[37] and we[38] have demonstrated EBNA and EBV genome, respectively, in Burkitt-like lymphomas of patients with AIDS. Of importance, in the patient we studied with an EBV-carrying B cell lymphoma, elevated VCA and EA antibody titers were not found. Failure to make anti-EA antibodies was likely due to the immune deficiency.

Adding support to the association of EBV with Burkitt-like lymphomas in patients with AIDS has been the occurrence of reciprocal translocations involving chromosomes 8 and 14 and 8 and 22 in tumor cells from these patients.[38-40] The breakpoints were on chromosome 8 at band q24 where c-myc oncogene resides and on chromosome 14 at band q32 where the heavy chain Ig locus resides. These translocations are identical to findings in non-AIDS-associated Burkitt lymphoma cases. Translocation and approximation of the active Ig locus with c-myc is thought to lead to deregulation of c-myc expression.[41]

Evidence is mounting that enhanced chromosomal breakage in lymphocytes occurs in patients at risk for AIDS. Computer-assisted image analysis of lymphoid cells in pre-AIDS and AIDS shows increased polyploidy. These changes are comparable to other viral induced diseases such as papillomatosis.[31,42] These findings probably signal interference of cellular divison by virus or other factors. Also, Manolov et al.[43] have demonstrated structural aberrations in healthy, promiscuous homosexuals as well as those with lymphadenomegaly. These aberrations including breaks and reciprocal translocations characteristic of malignancies seem to disappear in patients with AIDS. We have speculated that viral infection leads to these breakpoints and translocations.

Perhaps HTLV-III as well as EBV could be important in evoking these changes. Death of cells with chromosomal aberrations could lead to the disappearance of chromosomal aberrations. Concurrently, T4 populations become depleted, possibly due to HTLV-III infection yielding lysis of the cells. We have stated earlier that the prevailing idea is that a single agent (i.e., HTLV-III) is responsible for AIDS,[44] however, we think that deleterious immune responses to CMV, EBV, and antigens from other sources[30] could suppress immunity and thereby prepare the host for a final insult.

Hypothesis: Interaction between EBV and HTLV-III in the Induction of AIDS

Polymicrobial infections involving virtually every microbe and organ system are associated with pre-AIDS and AIDS in male homosexuals. Noted earlier, nearly 100% of the male homosexuals we have studied have been EBV seropositive and all but a few were seropositive for CMV. Hepatitis B virus seropositivity and antibodies to sexually transmitted infectious agents were found in the vast majority of patients.

The humoral limb of immunity is perturbed in pre-AIDS and AIDS patients. Well known is the hyperimmunoglobulinemia accompanying infectious diseases such as infectious mononucleosis. CMV, commonly infecting patients with AIDS can in addition to EBV, also be a polyclonal activator of B cells.[45] Stimulation of Ig synthesis occurs even though the patients have an increased number of suppressor T cells. This paradox of acute infectious mononucleosis is also observed in patients with AIDS. Lane et al.[46] have demonstrated elevated numbers of B cells spontaneously secreting immunoglobulin, decreased B cell proliferative responses to T cell-independent B cell mitogens, and qualitatively deficient helper T cells. These features suggest an in-vivo polyclonal activation of B cells reflecting the B cell hyperactivity-hyperimmunoglobulinemia and possibly explain the autoantibody production. Noted earlier, EBV[13] and CMV[45] are polyclonal activators of B cells in-vitro. Furthermore, Notkin's group[47] have demonstrated the production of IgM isotype autoantibodies from lymphoblastoid cell lines established in-vitro from patients with autoimmune disorders. Some of the autoimmune disorders of patients with AIDS and pre-AIDS could be derived in-vivo due to uncontrolled B cell activation by EBV and CMV. Patients with acute infectious mononucleosis usually show anti-neutrophil antibodies and neutropenia.[14] The neutropenia in the male homosexuals could be due to a similar mechanism or from CMV or other infections. In addition to EBV and CMV as polyclonal B cell activators,[13] it is probable that other microbes could also evoke a similar immune response after they are showered into the portal blood stream during anal intercourse.

Our hypothesis must also account for thymic defects in the patients.[4] Thymic epithelial destruction, elevated thymosin alpha, immaturity of T cell populations and immunoregulatory disturbances are also important aspects of the immunopathogenesis of AIDS. These are discussed elsewhere in this volume by Goldstein.

Montagnier's group at the Pasteur Institute has recently reported that infection of EBV infected lymphoblastoid B cell lines with lymphadenopathy-associated virus (LAV) leads to a markedly enhanced production of the retrovirus.[48] We[49] have established an infected EBV- and HLTV-III-carrying B lymphoblastoid cell line from a male homosexual (Figure 1). It has been known for more than a decade that retroviruses can become reactivated when immune stimulation occurs. For example, murine retroviruses can become very active during graft vs. host disease.[50] We propose that EBV and CMV and various immune responses activate both B and T cells in-vivo and thus may allow HTLV-III to infect

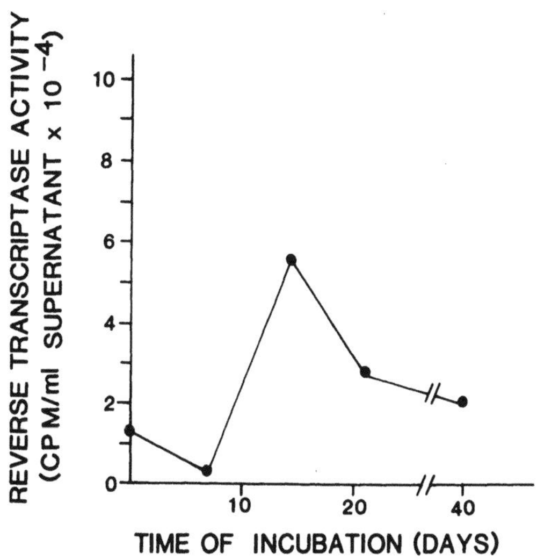

Fig. 1. Detection of a retrovirus in cultured peripheral blood lymphocytes from a lymphadenopathy patient. Peripheral blood lymphocytes were isolated by Ficoll/Isopaque gradient centrifugation and cultured first in the presence of PHA and then with interleukin-2. Cell supernatants were collected at the designated time, concentrated and analyzed for reverse transcriptase activity (RT). The poly(A)-dependent DNA polymerase activity (RT) was measured in 50 1 of 50 mMTrisx HCl, pH 7.5/5mM DTT/100 mM KCl/10 mM $MgCl_2$/10 M (^3H)dTTP/ 0.1% Triton X-100 containing 2 μg of poly(A), 0.4 μg of oligo$[dT]_{12-18}$ and 20 μl of the concentrated supernatant. The established cell line expressed B-1 monoclonal surface marker and no T cell markers. The cells were EBV genome positive. The presence of a retrovirus in the cell line was confirmed by electron microscopy.

stimulated B cells as well as T helper cells. The productive infection by HTLV-III in the simultaneously infected B cells may allow spread of the virus throughout the immune system. Helper T cells would then become extensively infected resulting in their lysis and depletion. This hypothesis is currently being tested in our laboratories.[51]

SUMMARY

We have reviewed the biologic characteristics, immune responses, and diverse array of diseases occurring from Epstein-Barr virus infections in immune deficient patients. We have summarized possible roles of the virus in the risk groups for AIDS. Data is convincing that EBV is responsible for some of the cases of lymphadenomegaly and Burkitt-like, non-Hodgkin's lymphomas in patients with pre-AIDS and AIDS. A hypothesis has been proposed wherein EBV and other stimulants of B and T cells allow productive infection by the retrovirus and spread of HTLV-III throughout the helper T cell populations.

ACKNOWLEDGMENTS

This work was supported in part by PHS grant CA30196 (DTP) and CA37465 (DJV) awarded by the National Cancer Institute DHHS, the Lymphoproliferative-AIDS Research Fund, and the Nebraska State Department of Health LB506.

REFERENCES

1. F. Barre-Sinoussi, J.-C. Chermann, F. Rey, T. Nugeyre, S., Chamaret, J. Gruest, C. Dauguet, and C. Axler-Blin, Isolation of a T-lymphotropic retrovirus from a patient at risk for acquired immune deficiency syndrome (AIDS). Science 220:868 (1983).
2. P. Pattengale, R.W. Smith, and P. Gerber, Selective transformation of B lymphocytes by E.B. virus. Lancet 2:93 (1973).
3. G.P.A. Rice, R.D. Schrier, and M.B.A. Oldstone, Cytomegalovirus infects human lymphocytes and monocytes: virus expression is restricted to immediate-early gene products. Proc. Natl. Acad. Sci. USA 81:6134 (1984).
4. D.T. Purtilo, H. Lipscomb, S. Harada, J. Hayes, G. Manolov, Y. Manolova, S. Witkin, and J. Sonnabend, Etiological factors in the induction of acquired immune deficiency syndrome (AIDS), in: "Clinical Laboratory Molecular Analyses: New Strategies in Autoimmunity, Cancer and Virology," R. Nakamura, ed., Grune and Stratton, New York (in press).
5. W. Henle, G. Henle, and E.T. Lennette, The Epstein-Barr virus, Sci. Am. 241:48 (1979).
6. J.W. Sixbey, J.G. Nedrud, N. Raab-Traub, R.A. Hanes, and J.S. Pagano, Epstein-Barr virus replication in oropharyneal epithelial cells, N. Engl. J. Med. 310:1225 (1984).
7. H. Wolf, E. Wilnes, and S.G.J. Bayliss, Epstein-Barr virus: its site of persistence and its role in the development of carcinomas, in : "Modern Trends in Human Leukemia, IV," Neth et al, eds., Springer-Verlag, Heidelburg, Berlin (1981).
8. D.T. Purtilo, "Immune Deficiency and Cancer: Epstein-Barr Virus and Lymphoproliferative Malignancies," Plenum Press, New York (1984).
9. D.T. Purtilo, Immune deficiency predisposing to Epstein-Barr virus-induced lymphoproliferative diseases: the X-linked lymphoproliferative syndrome as a model, Adv. Cancer Res. 34:279 (1980).
10. D.T. Purtilo, Hypothesis: pathogenesis and phenotypes of an X-linked recessive lymphoproliferative syndrome, Lancet 2:882 (1976).
11. G. Tosato, I. Magrath, I. Koski, N. Dooley, and M. Blaese, Activation of suppressor T cells during Epstein-Barr-virus-induced infectious mononucleosis, N. Engl. J. Med. 301:1133 (1979).
12. J. Robinson, D. Smith, and J. Niederman, Plasmacytic differentiation of circulating Epstein-Barr virus-infected B lymphocytes during acute infectious mononucleosis, J. exp. Med. 153:235 (1981).
13. A. Rosen, P. Gergely, M. Jondal, G. Klein, and S. Britton, Polyclonal Ig production after Epstein-Barr virus infection in human lymphocytes in vitro, Nature 267:52 (1977).
14. R.T. Schooley, P. Densen, D. Harmon, D. Velzenstein, M.S. Hirsch, W. Henle, and S. Whitzman, Anti-neutrophil antibodies in infectious mononucleosis, Am. J. Med. 76:85 (1984).
15. J. Linder and D.T. Purtilo, Infectious mononucleosis, in: "Immune Deficiency and Cancer: Epstein-Barr Virus and Lymphoproliferative Malignancies," D.T. Purtilo, ed., Plenum Press, New York, p. 11 (1984).
16. D.T. Purtilo, Immunopathology of X-linked lymphoproliferative syndrome, Immunol. Today 4:291 (1983).

17. D.T. Purtilo, K. Sakamoto, V. Barnabei, J. Seeley, T. Bechtold, G. Rogers, J. Yetz, and S. Harada, Epstein-Barr virus-induced diseases in males with the X-linked lymphoproliferative syndrome (XLP), Am. J. Med. 73:49 (1982).
18. D. Weisenburger and D.T. Purtilo, Failures in immunological control of EB virus infection: fatal infectious mononucleosis, in, "The Epstein-Barr Virus: Recent Advances," M.A. Epstein and B.G. Achong, eds., William Heinemann Medical Books, Ltd., England, in press
19. S. Harada, T. Bechtold, and D.T. Purtilo, Cell-mediated immunity to Epstein-Barr virus (EBV) and natural killer (NK)-cell activity in X-linked lymphoproliferative syndrome, Int. J. Cancer 216: 739 (1982).
20. S. Argov, D. Johnson, M. Collins, H.S. Koren, H. Lipscomb, and D.T. Purtilo, Loss of natural killing (NK) activity but retention of lymphocyte mediated antibody-dependent cellular cytotoxicity (ADCC) in patients with the X-linked lymphoproliferative syndrome (XLP), submitted for publication.
21. A. Rubinstein,M. Sicklick, A. Gupta, L. Bernstein, N. Klein, E. Rubinstein, I. Spigland, L. Fruchter, N. Litman, H. Lee, and M. Hollander, Acquired immunodeficiency with reversed T4/T8 ratios in infants born to promiscuous and drug-addicted mothers, J. Am. Med. Assoc. 249:2325 (1983).
22. J. Oleske, A. Minnefor, R. Cooper, K. Thomas, A. dela Cruz, H. Ahdieh, I. Guerrero, V.V. Joski, and F. Desposito, Immune deficiency syndrome in children, J. Am. Med. Assoc. 249:2345 (1983).
23. R.J. McDonough, J.J. Madden, A. Falek, D.A. Shafer, M. Pline, D. Gordon, P. Bokos, J.C. Kuehnle, and J. Mendelson, Alteration of T and null lymphocyte frequencies in the peripheral blood of human opiate receptor sites on T lymphocytes, J. Immunol. 125:2539 (1980).
24. F. Gervais, C. Tsoukas, A. Fuks, and J. Shuster, Natural history of the AIDS related complex in hemophilia - relationships to Epstein-Barr virus, AIDS Res. 1:197 (1984).
25. Mobidity and Mortality Weekly Report, Update: acquired immuno-deficiency syndrome (AIDS) - United States, 32:688 (1984).
26. Morbidity and Mortality Weekly Report, Opportunistic infections and Kaposi's sarcoma among Haitians in the United States 31:353 (1982).
27. A.E. Pitchenik, M.A. Fischl, G.M. Dickinson, D.M. Becker, A.M. Fournier, M.T. O'Connell, R.M. Colton, and T.J. Spira, Opportunistic infections and Kaposi's sarcoma among Haitians: evidence of a new acquired immunodeficiency state. Ann. Intern. Med. 98:277 (1983).
28. R.B. Purtilo, J. Sonnabend, and D.T. Purtilo, Confidentiality, informed consent and untoward social consequences in research on a "new killer disease" (AIDS), Clin. Res. 31:462 (1983).
29. D.T. Purtilo and D.H. Connor, Fatal infections in protein-calorie malnourished children with thymolymphatic atrophy, Arch. Dis. Childh. 50:149 (1975).
30. J. Sonnabend, S. Witkin, and D.T. Purtilo, Acquired immunodeficiency syndrome, opportunistic infections, and malignancies in male homo-sexuals. A hypothesis of etiologic factors in pathogenesis, J. Am. Med. Assoc. 249:2370 (1983).
31. G.R.F. Krueger, W. Otten, M. Ortmann, L. Haussermann, C. Rasokat, K. Degenhardt, R. Hehlmann, H. Wolf, W. Auffermann, A. Bocking, and A. Ramon, Immunopathology of AIDS (acquired immune deficiency syndrome). Observations in 54 patients with pre-AIDS and AIDS. Path. Res. Pract. (in press) (1984).
32. H. Lipscomb, E. Tatsumi, S. Harada, J. Sonnabend, J. Wallace, J. Yetz, J. Davis, K. McClain, C. Metroka, R. Tubbs, and D.T. Purtilo, Epstein-Barr virus, chronic lymphadenomegaly, and lymphoma in male homosexuals with acquired immunodeficiency syndrome (AIDS). AIDS Res. 1:59 (1983).

33. M. Marmor, L. Laubenstein, D.C. William et al., Risk factors for Kaposi's sarcoma in homosexual men, Lancet 2:125 (1982).
34. R. DuBois, J. Seeley, S. Harada, M. Ballow, and D.T. Purtilo, Chronic Epstein-Barr virus infection and mononucleosis, Southern Med. J. 77:1376 (1984).
35. D.H. Crawford, I. Willard, I. Leiscu, and D.W. Wara, Epstein-Barr (EB) virus infection in homosexual men in London, Br. J. Vener. Dis. 60:258 (1984).
36. J.L. Ziegler, J.A. Beckstead, P.A. Volberding, D.I. Abrams, A.M. Levine, R.J. Lukes, P.S. Gill, R.L. Burkes, P.R. Meyer, C.E. Metroka, J. Mouradian, A. Morre, S.A. Riggs, J.J Butler, F.C. Cabanillas, E. Hersh, G.R. newell, L.J. Laubenstein, D. Knowles, C. Odajnyk, B. Raphael, B. Koziner, C. Urmacher, and B.D. Clarkson, Non-Hodgkin's lymphoma in 90 homosexual men. Relation to generalized lymphadenopathy and the acquired immunodeficiency syndrome, N. Engl. J. Med. 311:565 (1984).
37. J.L. Ziegler, R.C. Miner, E. Rosenbaum, E.T. Lennette, E. Shillitoe, C. Casavant, W.L. Drew, L. Mintz, J. Gershow, J. Greenspan, J. Beckstead, and K. Yamamoto, Outbreak of Burkitt's-like lymphoma in homosexual men, Lancet 2:631 (1982).
38. J.M. Petersen, R.R. Tubbs, R.A. Savage, L.C. Calabrese, M.R. Proffitt, Y. Manolova, G. Manolov, A. Schumaker, E. Tatsumi, K. McClain, and D.T. Purtilo, Small noncleaved B cell Burkitt-type lymphoma with chromosome t(8;14) translocation and carrying Epstein-Barr virus in a male homosexual with the acquired immune deficiency syndrome, Am. J. Med., in press (1984).
39. R.S.K. Chaganti, C. Suresh, B.K. Jhanwar, Z. Arlin, R. Mertelsmann, and B.D. Clarkson, Specific translocations characterize Burkitt's like lymphoma of homosexual men with the acquired immunodeficiency syndrome, Blood 61:1265 (1983).
40. I. Magrath, J. Erikson, J. Whang-Peng, H. Sieverts, G. Armstrong, D. Benjamin, T. Triche, O. Alabaster, and C.M. Croce, Synthesis of kappa light chains by cell lines containing an 8;22 chromosomal translocation derived from a male homosexual with Burkitt's lymphoma, Science 222:1094 (1983).
41. P. Leder, J. Battey, G. Lenoir, C. Moulding, W. Murphy, H. Potter, T. Steward, and R. Taub, Translocations among antibody genes in human cancer, Science 222:765 (1983).
42. W. Auffermann, G.R.F. Krueger, and A. Bocking, Chromatinverteilung und DNS-Gehalt bei AIDS als Zeichen viraler Infektion-Analyse durch DNA Bildzytometrie, Verh. Dtsch. Ges. Path. 68: (in press) (1984).
43. G. Manolov, Y. Manolova, J. Sonnabend, H. Lipscomb, and D.T. Purtilo, Chromosome aberrations in peripheral lymphocytes of promiscuous male homosexuals predisposed to acquired immune deficiency syndrome (AIDS), AIDS Res. 1:157 (1984).
44. A.S. Fauci, The acquired immune deficiency syndrome, J. Am. Med. Assoc. 249:2375 (1983).
45. L. Hutt-Fletcher, N. Balchandarn, and M.H. Elkins, B cell activation by cytomegalovirus, J. Exp. Med. 158:2171 (1983).
46. H.C. Lane, H. Masur, L.C. Edgar, G. Whalen, A.H. Rook, and A.S. Fauci, Abnormalities of B cell activation and immunoregulation in patients with the acquired immune deficiency syndrome, N. Engl. J. Med. 309:453 (1983).
47. C. Garzelli, F.E. Taub, J.E. Scharff, B.S. Prabhakar, F. Ginsberg-Gellner, and A.L. Notkins, Epstein-Barr virus-transformed lymphocytes produce monoclonal autoantibodies that react with antigens in multiple organs, J. Virol. 52:722 (1984).
48. L. Montagnier, J. Gruest, S. Chamaret, C. Dauguet, C. Axler, D. Guetard, M.T. Nugeyre, F. Barre-Sinoussi, J.-C. Chermann, D. Klatzmann, and J.C. Gluckman, Adaptation of lymphadenopathy-

associated virus (LAV) to replication in EBV-transformed B lymphoblastoid cell lines, Science 225:63 (1984).
49. D. Casareale, and D.J. Volsky, Isolation of EBV- and HTLV-III-carrying B cell lines from blood of patients with lymphoadenopathy and AIDS, submitted for publication.
50. R.S. Schwartz, Immunoregulation, oncogenic viruses, and malignant lymphomas, Lancet 2:1266 (1972).
51. D. Casareale, J. Sonnabend, F. Sinangil, D.T. Purtilo, and D.J. Volsky, Detection of retroviruses in blood of patients with acquired immune deficiency syndrome (AIDS)-related conditions and in healthy individuals from New York City, submitted for publication.

LONGITUDINAL IMMUNOLOGICAL STUDIES ON A COHORT OF INITIALLY SYMPTOM-FREE HOMOSEXUAL MEN IN LONDON WITH RESPECT TO HTLV-III SEROLOGY

A.J. Pinching, J.N. Weber, L.A. Rogers, E.L. Berrie, D.J. Jeffries and J.R.W. Harris

Departments of Immunology and Virology
St Mary's Hospital Medical School
and the Praed Street Clinic
LONDON W2, England

INTRODUCTION

In late 1981, when AIDS was becoming increasingly well-documented in the USA, we set up a study to examine cellular immmunity in symptom-free homosexuals in London. We felt that if AIDS did not develop, it would be of interest to determine why not, since the life-style of this community was known to be similar to that in New York. On the other hand, if the disease were indeed to develop, we had an important opportunity to study the background cellular immunological profile of sexually active gay men before the disease emerged; such a high-risk, low-incidence population was not as readily studied in the USA. It has since been shown that AIDS is an infectious disease caused by the novel retrovirus HTLV-III/LAV. An epidemic of this infection has occurred in the UK following that in the US by some three years. By December 1984 there had been 102 cases in the UK (35 at St Mary's), compared with 28 at the same time in 1983 and 7 at the end of 1982. Persistent generalised lymphadenopathy (PGL) has also increased over the same period: at the Praed Street Clinic, a large clinic for sexually transmitted diseases, we had seen a total of only 7 cases in 1982, but this had risen to 47 by the end of 1983 and to 150 at the present. A recent study on the prevalence of antibodies to HTLV-III in the UK (Cheingsong-Popov et al, 1984) has shown that 17% of symptom-free homosexuals were seropositive.

Our cohort of symptom-free homosexual men was recruited in 1982 and the first half of 1983, before the major rise in AIDS cases. They included persons attending the clinic for screening and volunteers from the community following articles in the gay press. This meant that diverse life-styles were represented. The immunological features of the cohort at recruitment have been described (Pinching et al, 1983); these showed a wide variety of abnormalities, including some that resembled those seen in AIDS. In November 1983 we reported data which indicated that some of the defects appeared to be transient (Pinching et al, 1984). We have now studied 110 homosexual men longitudinally, for 89 of whom we have data on HTLV-III serology. Serial studies on those who are now seropositive are not yet complete. In this preliminary analysis, we examine the cellular immunology profiles obtained longitudinally in relation to current HTLV-III serology and clinical course.

PATIENTS AND METHODS

Patients were recruited as above and answered an initial questionnaire about life-style and health. They were examined and screened for sexually transmitted and other disease. Blood was taken for immunological and virological studies. Delayed type hypersensitivity (DTH) skin tests were set up for Purified Protein Derivative, Candida albicans and Streptokinase/Streptodornase. They were read at 48-72 hours and 4mm or more of induration was taken as positive. Anergy was defined as negative results with all three antigens. Patients were followed up at intervals of 6-12 months with repeat questionnaires and immunological profiles at 12 months.

Lymphocyte counts were obtained from coulter and differential counts; the lower limit of normal was set at 1.5 x 10 /l. T cell subsets were defined using monoclonal antibody testing on freshly obtained separated cells with a suitable fluorescent second label. Leu 3a defined T "helper" cells and Leu 2a T "suppressor/cytotoxic" cells. Results were read on a fluorescence microscope or on the EPICS-V cell sorter/analyser. Results were expressed as total counts of the two subsets, with the lower limit of normal for Leu 3a having been previously established at 0.53 x 10 /l, and the upper limit
9
for Leu 2a being arbitrarily taken as 0.8 x 10 /l. Monocyte phagocytosis was estimated using Candida guilliermondii as target as previously described (Pinching et al, 1983), with 94% of the value of the simultaneous normal control as the lower limit of normal.

Antibodies to HTLV-III were detected in a membrane fluorescence assay using HTLV-III infected H9 cells kindly provided by Prof R Weiss and originally obtained from Dr R Gallo. Some results were obtained in the competitive radioimmunoassay of Cheingsong-Popov et al, 1984. Sera tested in both assays showed complete concordance. The most recent serum was tested for the present study.

RESULTS:

Of the original cohort of 110, 2 patients have developed AIDS (2%) and 18 PGL (17%); 3 of the latter had incomplete studies. Four of the PGL patients were seronegative, although in all other respects they resembled the seropositive subjects, and two of them were sexual contacts of AIDS patients. It seems likely that these subjects were seronegative despite active HTLV-III infection. The patients in whom clinical progression occurred will be analysed as a single group ("Progressive"). The seropositivity rate was 35% for the whole group of 89 in whom there are complete serial studies, and this rises to a presumed incidence of 39% HTLV-III infection if the four seronegative PGL patients are included.

In the following analysis (Table I), changes in lymphocytes and subsets, monocyte phagocytosis and DTH responses will be studied for three groups of subjects: symptom-free seronegative (H-ve)(54), symptom-free seropositive (H+ve)(18) and progressive (Prog)(17).

Table I: Serial Immunological Profile in 89 Symptom-Free Homosexual Men According to Serology or Progression

NB For each group, the percentage of subjects showing the given immunological features is shown.

Immunological results	H-ve	H+ve	Prog.
Lymphocytes (a)			
Normal throughout	70%	77%	59%
Developed lymphopenia	4%	11%	0%
Lymphopenia persisted	4%	6%	6%
Lymphopenia regressed	22%	6%	35%
T helper cells (Leu 3a) (b)			
Normal throughout	77%	71%	47%
Th-penia developed	10%	17%	20%
Th-penia persisted	0%	6%	13%
Th-penia regressed	13%	6%	20%
Th-penia ± sign. fall*	25%	67%	53%
T supp/cyto cells (Leu 2a) (c)			
Normal throughout	58%	25%	33%
Ts-osis developed	13%	37%	27%
Ts-osis persisted	6%	19%	7%
Ts-osis regressed	23%	19%	33%
Th/Ts (Leu 3a/Leu 2a) Ratio (d)			
Normal throughout	55%	18%	12%
Th/Ts fell	4%	35%	25%
Th/Ts persistently low	17%	35%	44%
Th/Ts normalised	24%	12%	19%
Monocyte Phagocytosis (e)			
Ever abnormal	28%	28%	47%
Delayed Type Hypersensitivity			
Persistently anergic	21%	59%	33%
Anergic at any time	28%	59%	33%

a) Lower limit of normal $1.5 \times 10^{9}/l$

b) Lower limit of normal $0.53 \times 10^{9}/l$

c) Upper limit of normal $0.8 \times 10^{9}/l$

d) Lower limit of normal 1.2

e) Lower limit of normal 94%C

* Persistently low T helpers or a fall of $0.3 \times 10^{9}/l$.

As can be seen from the Table, immunological abnormalities were commonly present in seronegative as well as in seropositive patients. In the case of the seronegative subjects, the HTLV-III antibody status is based on the most recent serum sample and therefore the changes can be assumed to be unrelated to HTLV-III infection; we appreciate that there may be a few false negatives but these cannot account for most of the abnormalities found. On the other hand, the seropositive subjects may have seroconverted between the first study and the present; so some at least of the changes may be related to seroconversion, while others may reflect serial changes occurring following infection in symptom-free subjects. A similar argument applies to the patients in whom progression was noted.

Lymphopenia was seen at some time during investigation in a similar proportion of those who were seropositive and seronegative but was more common among those who progressed. However, developing lymphopenia or persistent lymphopenia were more common among the seropositive subjects, while lymphopenia was more commonly transient among seronegative subjects. However, normalisation of lymphocyte count commonly accompanied the development of lymphadenopathy.

T helper cell depletion (Th-penia) was seen at some stage in as many seropositive as seronegative subjects, but was more common among those who progressed. Developing or persistent Th-penia were commoner among seropositive and progressive patients; normalisation of the Th count was seen in most of the seronegative subjects who showed an initial reduction. However, a significant proportion of patients who progressed showed a normalisation of the Th count as PGL developed. Among seropositive subjects and those who progressed either persistent Th-penia or a significant fall in Th count (even if this was still within the normal range) were common. In both of the subjects who developed AIDS, we observed a significant fall in Th within the normal range, only one of them eventually developing absolute Th depletion.

Changes in T suppressor/cytotoxic cells were common in all groups, especially in the seropositive and progressive groups. A rise in T suppressors, or persistently elevated Ts, was seen in most seropositive subjects but a significant proportion showed transient changes. Among seronegative subjects the elevation in Ts count was usually transient. A substantial number of those who developed PGL showed a normalisation of the Ts count coincident with the development of PGL.

As would be expected from the above, changes in the Th/Ts ratio were common in all groups, although more frequent in the seropositive and progressive groups. Falling or persistently low Th/Ts ratios were more common in the latter two groups. Nevertheless, 45% of seronegative subjects had an abnormal ratio at some stage.

Monocyte phagocytic abnormalities were found in all groups but especially among those who progressed. The abnormalities were often transient, many being seen only at the first investigation. Anergy to the three recall antigens was found more frequently among seropositive and progressive patients but there was a significant incidence of anergy among the seronegative group, in some of whom it was transient.

DISCUSSION:

We have reported on longitudinal studies of cellular immunity in a population of initially symptom-free subjects recruited from a high-risk, low-incidence population of male homosexuals. The results indicate some of tie difficulties inherent in the interpretation of isolated immunological studies on sexually active gay men. They indicate that, even in the absence of HTLV-III infection, such subjects may show a number of the defects in cellular immunity, including those that are characteristic of AIDS. The diverse abnormalities among the seropositive subjects who remained well, and in those who developed PGL or AIDS during the period of study, further indicate the varied phenotypic responses that may follow HTLV-III infection. While some of these could have been predicted from a knowledge of the changes seen in AIDS (Seligmann et al, 1984) and of the tropism of the virus for cells of the helper phenotype (Dalgleish et al, 1984), others were quite distinct. Specifically this includes the increased numbers of T suppressor/cytotoxic phenotype that were seen in a substantial proportion of infected subjects; this resembles the early response seen in other viral infections such as those with cytomegalovirus and Epstein-Barr virus. Many of the immunological abnormalities found on initial study of patients who subsequently developed PGL resolved as the lymphadenopathy arose. It is especially important to bear these early changes in mind when considering the ones that are seen after the development of PGL, other AIDS-associated syndromes or AIDS, since the latter clearly occur relatively late in terms of the evolution of immune abnormalities following retrovirus infection.

Further study of this group of subjects may help to indicate whether or not the immunological features associated with the acquisition of HTLV-III infection have any influence on outcome. It will be particularly important to determine which subjects have seroconverted while under study; this will not only be to define the earliest changes following the acquisition of the infection but also to determine whether the prior immune state had an influence on the course of infection. It may be that the different immunological features following HTLV-III infection reflect differing phenotypic responses to that infection with different prognostic significance. Alternatively they may reflect differing stages in the evolution of a slowly progressive disorder. Another possible interpret- ation is that some or all of the changes seen in seropositive subjects are a reflection of intercurrent events such as other viral infections in HTLV-III infected subjects, infections that may not only influence the immune parameters under study but may also have a critical bearing on the subsequent development of disease or possibly of protective immunity. Only by further longitudinal study of such a cohort can these possible inter- pretations be honed down; it is our hope that such studies will clarify the way in which the novel lymphotropic retrovirus interacts with its host and the factors which affect the clinical expression of infection.

ACKOWLEDGEMENTS:

We wish to express our gratitude to our many colleagues - especially David Houghton, Owrang Moshtael and Di Flowers - and to our subjects, without whose unstinting cooperation this study could not have been done.

REFERENCES:

Cheingsong-Popov, R.,Weiss, R.A., Dalgleish, A., Tedder, R.S., Shanson, D.C., Jeffries D.J., Ferns, R.B., Briggs, E.M., Weller, I.V.D., Mitton,S., Adler, M.W., Farthing C., Lawrence, A.G., Gazzard, B.G., Weber, J., Harris, J.R.W., Pinching, A.J., Craske, J. and Barbara, J.A.J., 1984, Prevalence of antibody to human T-lymphotropic virus type III in AIDS and AIDS-risk patients in Britain, Lancet, ii;477.

Dalgleish, A.G., Beverley, P.C.L., Clapham, P., Crawford, D.H., Greaves, M.J. and Weiss, R.A., 1984, The CD4 (T4) antigen is an essential component of the receptor for the AIDS retrovirus (HTLV-3), Nature, 312;

Pinching, A.J., McManus, T.J., Jeffries D.J., Moshtael, O., Donaghy, M., Parkin, J.M., Munday, P.E. and Harris J.R.W., 1983, Studies of cellular immunity in male homosexuals in London, Lancet, ii;126.

Pinching A.J., Weber, J., Rogers, L.A., Jeffries D.J. and Harris, J.R.W., 1984, A longitudinal study of cellular immunity in male homosexuals in London, Annals of New York Academy of Sciences, 437; (in press).

Seligmann, M., Chess, L., Fahey, J.L., Fauci, A.S., Lachmann, P.J., L'Age Stehr, J., Ngu, J., Pinching, A.J., Rosen, F.S., Spira, T.J. and Wybran, J., 1984, AIDS - An immunologic reevaluation, New England Journal of Medicine, 311;1286.

LYMPHADENOPATHY: END-POINT PRODROME?

UPDATE OF A 36-MONTH PROSPECTIVE STUDY

Donald I. Abrams, Timothy Mess and Paul A. Volberding

San Francisco General Hospital
California 94110

In contrast to the situation in London described by Pinching, San Francisco physicians were faced with the challenge of persistent lymphadenopathy in homosexual men even before the AIDS epidemic had been defined(1). Although the initial cases of the lymphadenopathy syndrome were first appreciated in 1979, the prospective natural history study in our clinic was only initiated in November 1981(2). The 200 patients enrolled in this study clearly do not constitute the entirety of lymphadenopathy patients in San Francisco. Since the lymphadenopathy syndrome is not reportable to the Centers for Disease Control or the City Health Department, estimates of the number of men affected in the San Francisco area are difficult to obtain. As part of a case control study of 150 of our first AIDS patients, Moss and the Epidemiology group at San Francisco General Hospital interviewed and examined 300 matched controls(3). One hundred fifty participants were neighborhood controls, matched by age, race and socio-economic status to patients residing in the vicinity. One hundred fifty further controls were obtained from the municipal venereal disease clinic, also matched as closely as possible to cases. A concurrent study evaluated 150 sexual partners of documented AIDS patients. As part of this evaluation, the subjects underwent physical examination performed by physicians in clinic. Moss' results indicate that 16% of the neighborhood controls, 23% of venereal disease clinic controls, and 45% of the sexual partners of AIDS patients have palpable lymphadenopathy on examination which would meet criteria for inclusion into the lymphadenopathy syndrome cohort(4). A recent estimate suggests that the male homosexual population of San Francisco approaches 70,000(5). These figures tend to confirm speculations that the lymphadenopathy syndrome is approximately ten times more prevalent in homosexual men in San Francisco than full-blown AIDS.

The physical finding of generalized lymphadenopathy itself probably represents a nonspecific manifestation of infection with the AIDS retrovirus. The differential diagnosis of lymphadenopathy in risk groups includes neoplastic and infectious etiologies (see Table I). Kaposi's sarcoma may present in a purely lymphadenopathic form without mucocutaneous lesions. Similarly, nodal involvement with Kaposi's sarcoma may be seen in patients with cutaneous manifestation of the disease. Some patients with Kaposi's sarcoma have lymph node biopsies which are indistinguishable from the follicular hyperplasia seen in patients with the lymphadenopathy syndrome(6). Lymphomas, both Hodgkin's and non-Hodgkin's, have been seen with increased frequency in the male homosexual population in San Francisco(7,8).

Lymphadenopathy has also been appreciated in AIDS patients presenting with opportunistic infections. Approximately 50% of patients diagnosed with Pneumocystis pneumonia in our clinic have lymphadenopathy palpable on initial evaluation. The Pneumocystis infection itself is not directly responsible for the lymphadenopathy in these cases. Infections in which actual micro-organisms have been cultured or identified in the node microscopically include Mycobacterial diseases, either typical tuberculosis or avium-intracellulare(9). Disseminated coccidioidomycosis has been diagnosed by lymph node biopsy in a risk group patient(10). Toxoplasmosis may cause generalized lymphadenopathy with characteristic histopathologic changes noted on lymph node biopsy(11). However, toxoplasmosis in AIDS patients is more frequently diagnosed on biopsy of central nervous system lesions as opposed to lymph node pathology(12).

The miscellaneous causes of diffuse lymphadenopathy in AIDS-related risk groups have included angio-immunoblastic lymphadenopathy and angiofollicular hyperplasia or Castleman's disease(13,14). The particular subset of lymphadenopathy patients that is being followed prospectively by many of the groups attending this conference are those with benign reactive adenopathy. Patients entered into our prospective natural history study of the lymphadenopathy syndrome have had at least six months of persistent adenopathy prior to entry(2). Lymph nodes must be present in two or more extra-inguinal sites with nodes greater than 1 cm. in diameter. Patients enrolled may or may not suffer from systemic symptoms. Non-AIDS-related causes of lymphadenopathy have been previously excluded by the patient's referring physician.

Table I: Differential Diagnosis of AIDS-Related Lymphadenopathy

<u>Neoplasms</u>

- Kaposi's sarcoma
- Non-Hodgkin's lymphoma (usually B cell origin)
- Hodgkin's disease

<u>Infections</u>

- Pneumocystis carinii pneumonia
- Mycobacterium avium-intracellulare or tuberculosis
- Coccidioides immitis
- Toxoplasmosis

<u>Miscellaneous</u>

- Angioimmunoblastic lymphadenopathy
- Angiofollicular hyperplasia (Castleman's disease)
- Lymphadenopathy syndrome (reactive hyperplasia)

Approximately one-half of our cohort of patients have undergone lymph node biopsies. All but two of the specimens have demonstrated a pattern of florid follicular hyperplasia. Marked expansion of the germinal centers impinging into the paracortex is noted. In addition, the paracortical region is involved with increased plasma cells, immunoblasts and vascularity(2,15,16). The pattern of involution described by Metroka has not been appreciated in our population(17,18).

Even before the sero-epidemiologic studies confirmed that the putative AIDS retrovirus was involved in the pathogenesis of the lymphadenopathy syndrome, many similarities between men with persistent lymphadenopathy syndrome and patients with bona fide AIDS had been identified. Demographic profiles of the two groups are nearly identical. First noted to be a common problem in the male homosexual population, persistent generalized lymphadenopathy was initially named the "Gay Lymph Node Syndrome". This has become a misnomer as the lymphadenopathy syndrome has subsequently been identified in all other AIDS risk groups(19,20,21,22,23,24,25). The geographic distribution of the lymphadenopathy syndrome also closely parallels that of AIDS. Cases were first recognized in New York, San Francisco and Los Angeles and have been subsequently appreciated in areas that were not initially endemic such as London and Atlanta (1,26,27). In questioning the 200 patients in our cohort as to the date of onset of their lymphadenopathy, all but six have stated that they developed their adenopathy since 1979 with the curve of onset dates roughly paralleling the increasing incidence of AIDS.

The symptoms that our patients describe are also reminiscent of those seen in patients with the full-blown acquired immunodeficiency syndrome. Thirty percent of patients are completely asymptomatic(28). Among the remainder, 50% experienced night sweats, fever and/or fatigue. Weight loss was described by one-third of the group. Another third of the patients complained of weight gain since the onset of their lymphadenopathy. Most patients attributed this to fatigue which forced them to abandon previous programs of physical exercise.

The lymph nodes are generally described as being non-tender. They wax and wane in size. Emotional stress, extreme fatigue, and the use of various illicit substances including marijuana, cocaine and nitrites have been described as causing the lymph nodes to increase in size. Abstinence from sexual activities, from drug use, and treatment with various antibiotics including tetracycline, erythromycin and anti-amoeba therapy have all been reported to cause transient decreases in the size of the nodes. In the group of patients with immune thrombocytopenia who also demonstrated peripheral lymphadenopathy, lymph nodes completely disappeared when patients were treated with high dose steroid therapy(29). Adenopathy recurred during tapering.

The review of systems of lymphadenopathy patients reveals that this group suffers from multiple non-life-threatening yet annoying infections. (See Table II). As described in Gottlieb's group, our patients also suffer from numerous skin infections(30). Tinea pedis, often unilateral and severe with nail involvement, is commonly seen.

Tinea cruris and corporis are appreciated less frequently. Lymphadenopathy patients have developed bullous impetigo in the groin and axilla. Warts are not only present in the perianal and genital regions but also on the oral mucosa. The Greenspans of the Department of Oral Medicine at the University of California San Francisco, have defined the wart-like lesion of the tongue, hairy leukoplakia, seen in a number of our lymphadenopathy patients(31). Other frequent infections encountered in the lymphadenopathy cohort include non-streptococcal pharyngitis, acute and chronic bacterial sinusitis, and intestinal parasites. The complaint of loose stool, often coated with mucous, has been evaluated in this group by doing routine ova and parasite evaluation on all patients in the lymphadenopathy protocol. Eighty percent of the cohort, regardless of symptomatology, have tested positive for an intestinal parasite. These include both potential pathogens and "non-pathogens" which should be considered as undesirable bowel inhabitants in this immunocompromised population.

Physical examination reveals lymph nodes present in axillary and inguinal regions in nearly 100% of the patients examined. The posterior cervical node is the one most frequently described as first noted by the patient. One-third of the cohort describe a flu-like illness prior to noting their adenopathy. The remaining two-thirds, however, oftentimes detected their posterior cervical lymph node on casual self examination. Other unusual sites for lymphadenopathy found on physical examination in these patients include epitrochlear nodes, usually only enlarged in secondary syphilis or non-Hodgkin's lymphoma, and the pre and posterior auricular nodes. The average number of node groups enlarged in our patients, counting right and left sides separately, is ten. Therefore, it is not difficult to appreciate the lymphadenopathy syndrome on physical examination. Patients presenting with a single isolated lymph node or two contiguous groups enlarged warrant immediate biopsy to rule out the possible presence of an underlying lymphomatous process.

Table II: Review of Systems in the Lymphadenopathy Syndrome

NODES:	Pain Bulk symptoms Nerve compression	ENT:	Sinus congestion Pharyngitis Herpes labialis Thrush Hairy leukoplakia
SKIN:	Tinea Onychomycosis. Impetigo Condylomata Herpes zoster Acne	GI:	Loose stool Perirectal eruptions
		CNS:	Headaches Anxiety/depression Distal neuropathy

Approximately one-third of patients evaluated have palpable spleens on physical examination. However, on performing abdominal CT scans on a smaller cohort of these patients, splenic enlargement was demonstrated in 75% of the group studied(32). Radiologists at San Francisco General Hospital have described a triad of findings on abdominal CT scan including splenomegaly, retroperitoneal lymphadenopathy, and thickening of the rectal mucosa consistent with a chronic proctitis in lymphadenopathy patients. The retroperitoneal nodes, found in 86% of lymphadenopathy patients, are generally small but increased in number when compared to controls. Despite the fact that these patients demonstrate lymphadenopathy above and below the diaphragm and intra-abdominally, chest X-rays in patients with the benign reactive syndrome are generally negative for hilar or mediastinal adenopathy(33). When thoracic adenopathy is appreciated, further workup should be entertained to pursue the diagnosis of a possible opportunistic infection or occult malignancy.

In our series, patients with benign reactive lymphadenopathy generally have normal complete blood counts including platelets and erythrocyte sedimentation rates. This is in contrast to reports from some of the other investigators participating in this conference(30,34). The serum chemistry panel is remarkable for a mild increase in total protein. Even in the absence of an elevated protein, serum protein electropheresis has demonstrated a polyclonal increase in the gamma globulin fraction in two-thirds of our patients. This reflects the B-cell hyperplasia that we see histologically on the lymph node biopsy. Isolated B-cells have been demonstrated to secrete immunoglobulin spontaneously at a level ten times greater than B-cells from control populations(35,36). In evaluating quantitative immunoglobulins, the predominant increase has been found in the IgG isotype. However, there is a statistically significant increase in IgA, IgM and IgE when compared to healthy homosexuals(37). Extremely elevated IgAs have been found mainly in patients with Pneumocystis pneumonia(38). About one-quarter of our patients demonstrate the presence of an antinuclear antibody, usually of low titer and in a diffuse pattern.

T-lymphycyte subsets demonstrate the reversed helper-to-suppressor ratio which has become a sine qua non of the acquired immunodeficiency syndrome. The average helper-to-suppressor ratio in our lymphadenopathy patients is 0.7. Two-thirds of the patients have a concomitant decrease in the OKT4 population and an increase in the OKT8 population. The remaining third showed decreased helper cells with normal suppressor cells. All of the patients demonstrate depletion of the T-helper cell population.

The complete immunologic profile of the lymphadenopathy syndrome demonstrates abnormalities in humoral as well as cell mediated immunity. Although we call the entire syndrome one of "immune deficiency", the lymphadenopathy cohort demonstrates frank immune dysregulation. There is a hypergammaglobulinemia in conjunction with depleted helper T-cells and defects in cell-mediated immunity demonstrated functionally by impaired mitogen responses and responses to recall antigens. The presence of the increased acid labile alpha interferon and decreased interleukin-2 production in lymphadenopathy patients have also been reported(39,40).

This prospective natural history study was initiated in November 1981. Thirty-six months of follow-up have been obtained on patients initially enrolled. The mean duration of follow-up in the cohort is 22 months. By the end of the first year of the study, none of the 70 patients enrolled had progressed to develop frank AIDS. By November 1983, 4 out of our 200 patients or 2% had evolved. At the present time, 14 of 200 patients have developed AIDS, 3 of whom have died. This mortality rate roughly parallels the San Francisco experience of an approximate one year average life span following an AIDS diagnosis(41). AIDS diagnoses which the lymphadenopathy patients have developed are listed in Table III. Two patients have developed Kaposi's sarcoma alone. The remaining 3 Kaposi's sarcoma patients have also been diagnosed with opportunistic infections. One patient developed 3 opportunistic infections in the year preceding his Kaposi's sarcoma. The other 2 patients were diagnosed with opportunistic infections following their Kaposi's sarcoma. Eleven instances of opportunistic infections have been reported in the patients progressing to AIDS. The most

Table III: Aids Diagnosed in Evolved Lymphadenopathy Syndrome

Kaposi's sarcoma	5
KS alone	2
KS, then OI	2
OI, then KS	1
Opportunistic Infection	11
Pneumocystis pneumonia	7
Cryptococcal meningitis	2
Mycobacterial disease	2
Cryptosporidium	1
Candida esophagitis	1
Lymphoma	1

common infection has been Pneumocystis pneumonia. One patient developed disseminated Mycobacterium tuberculosis. Another had disseminated Mycobacterium avium-intracellulare. An aggresssive B-cell lymphoma developed in one patient who expired within 2 weeks of diagnosis.

The clinical features of the 14 patients who evolved are seen in Table IV. The mean age of this subset of the cohort was 33 years, identical to that of the entire group. The mean duration of lymphadenopathy prior to the development of AIDS has been 29 months. These patients have been followed for a mean of 16 months in clinic. Constitutional symptoms, including fatigue, fever, night sweats and weight loss, were seen in 9 of the 14 patients at the time of their initial clinic evaluation. Three other patients developed constitutional symptoms during follow-up prior to their AIDS diagnosis. Two of our patients were diagnosed with AIDS at facilities outside the San Francisco Bay Area so complete details of their course prior to the AIDS diagnosis are unavailable. However, 10 of the 12 patients followed through their development of AIDS have experienced a decrease in the size of their peripheral lymphadenopathy, often to the point of disappearance.

Table IV: Clinical Features of the 14 Evolved LNS Patients

Age AIDS diagnosis	33 (21-47)
Months LNS prior to AIDS	29 (14-57)
Constitutional sx initially	9/14
Constitutional sx at AIDS Dx	12/14
Decreased lymphadenopathy	10/12

Various laboratory parameters have been suggested as factors that might be potentially predictive of which lymphadenopathy patients are at greatest risk to transform to AIDS. Studies have suggested that follicular involution or reversed helper-to-suppressor lymphocyte ratios within the actual lymph node specimen might be predictive(42). Other groups have found the presence of the HLA-DR5 marker to be of prognostic significance(43,44). The presence of acid labile alpha interferon has been described as a particularly sensitive assay which may define patients at risk to develop AIDS(45). Our study has demonstrated that relatively simple clinical and laboratory findings can be very predictive with regards to risk of progression(46) (see Table V). Antecedent thrush is perhaps the most significant finding with 10 of the 12 followed patients that developed AIDS demonstrating oral Candida either at initial presentation or antecedent to the ultimate diagnosis of their opportunistic infection or malignancy. This compares to only 10% of the stable cohort. Elevated erythrocyte sedimentation rates also appear to be predictive. A peripehral cytopenia also places the patient in the group with greater probability of progressing to AIDS. Patients referred to our clinic for evaluation of lymphadenopathy who demonstrate marked anemia, leukopenia, or moderate thrombocytopenia in association with an elevated erythrocyte sedimentation rate are not automatically included in the cohort of men with stable generalized lymphadenopathy. Instead these patients are aggressively evaluated from the outset for possible occult opportunistic infection or malignancy. Other centers evaluating lymphadenopathy patients include this subset in their natural history studies. This partially explains our lower incidence of progression to bona fide AIDS since these patients are diagnosed with an AIDS infection or malignancy prior to ever entering the stable cohort.

Table V: Clinical and Labortory Features of LNS Patients Evolved to AIDS Compared to Frequency of Abnormalities in the 200 Member Cohort

	AIDS	COHORT	SIGNIFICANCE*
Antecedent thrush	10/12	10%	p<.0001
Elevated sed rate	7/12	14%	p=.00081
Mild thrombocytopenia	5/14	8%	p=.0019
Leukopenia	5/14	6%	p=.0022
Anemia	3/14	5%	p=.043
History of Herpes Zoster	3/14	3%	p=.015
Hypocholesterolemia	4/14	20%	p=0.32

*Calculated by one-sided p value

Hypocholesterolemia has been noted in a number of patients with opportunistic infections, particularly Pneumocystis pneumonia. One of the lymphadenopathy patients had a normal cholesterol value at the time of his initial clinic evalution. However, by the time he developed Kaposi's sarcoma his serum cholesterol had fallen to 70 mg/dl in the absence of evident malnutrition. Although it appeared that hypocholesterolemia might be predictive for lymphadenopathy patients who would ultimately develop AIDS, the difference between the evolving patients and the stable cohort is not significant. Prior history of a herpes zoster infection is statistically significant in discriminating the subset of patients who have gone on to develop AIDS.

As recently as two years ago it was still necessary to attempt to convince the medical community that the syndrome of persistent generalized lymphadenopathy in homosexual men was, in fact, related to the newly described AIDS epidemic. However, with the advent of sero-epidemiologic studies and the identification of the putative AIDS retrovirus, most are now convinced that the lymphadenopathy syndrome is in fact an AIDS-related condition(47,48,49,50). Lymphadenopathy itself is probably a nonspecific physical finding common in AIDS and AIDS-related disorders most likely secondary to infection with the lymphotropic retrovirus. A subset of patients with a benign course and normal laboratory values is at low risk to develop major manifestations of AIDS. Simple clinical and laboratory findings may predict progression from the lymphadenopathy syndrome to the more malignant manifestations of acquired immunodeficiency.

REFERENCES

1. A. J. Pinching, Longitudinal immunological studies on a cohort of homosexual men in London with respect to HTLV III/LAV serology. This volume.

2. D. I. Abrams, B. J. Beckstead, J. H. Casavant C., and W. L. Drew. Persistent diffuse lymphadenopathy in homosexual men: Endpoint or prodrome? Ann Int Med, 100:801 (1984).

3. D. Osmond, A. R. Moss, P. Bachetti, P. Volberding, F. Barre-Sinoussi, J. and C. Chermann. A case-control study of risk factors for AIDS in San Francisco, International Conference on Acquired Immunodeficiency Syndrome (AIDS), Atlanta, GA (1985).
4. A. R. Moss, D. Osmond, P. Bachetti, D. Abrams, F. Barre-Sinnoussi and J. C. Chermann. One year followup of men exposed to AIDS in San Francisco, International Conference on Acquired Immunodeficiency Syndrome (AIDS), Atlanta, GA (1985).
5. L. Bye. Research and Decisions Corporation telephone survey for the San Francisco AIDS Foundation, International Conference on Acquired Immunodeficiency Syndrome (AIDS), Atlanta, GA (1985).
6. W. E. Finkbeiner, B. M. Egbert, J. R. Groundwater and R. W. Sagebiel. Kaposi's sarcoma in young homosexual men, Arch Pathol Lab Med 106:261 (1982).
7. J. L. Ziegler, J. A. Beckstead, P. A. Volberding, D. I. Abrams, A. M. Levine, R. J. Lukes et al. Non-Hodgkin's lymphoma in 90 homosexual men: Relationship to generalized lymphadenopathy and acquired immuno-deficiency syndrome (AIDS, New Engl J Med 311:565 (1984).
8. S. L. Schoeppel, R. T. Hoppe, R. F. Dorfman et al. AIDS and Hodgkin's disease, in: "Frontiers of Radiation Therapy and Oncology - Cancer and AIDS", Vol. 19, J. M. Vaeth, ed., Karger Publishing Co., Basal, pp 66-73, (1985).
9. M. L. Freeman and G. H. Talbot. Nongranulomatous mycobacterial lymphadenitis in homosexual patients. Laboratory Investigation 48:27A (abstract) (1983).
10. D. I. Abrams, M. Robia, W. Blumenfeld, J. Simonson., M. B. Cohen, and W. K. Hadley. Disseminated coccidioido-mycosis in AIDS, New Engl J Med 310:986 (1984).
11. H. L. Joachim. Toxoplasma lymphadenitis, in: "Lymph Node Biopsy", J. B. Lippincott Co., Philadelphia, Pa (1985).
12. B. J. Luft, R. G. Brooks, F. K. Conley, R. E. McCabe and J. S. Remington. Toxoplasmic encephalitis in patients with acquired immune deficiency syndrome, JAMA 252:913 (1984).
13. W. Blumenfeld and J. H. Beckstead. Angioimmunoblastic lymphadenopathy with dysproteinemia in homosexual men with acquired immune deficiency syndrome, Arch Pathol Lab Med 107:567 (1983).
14. N. A. Lachant, L. A. Leung, N. C. J. Sun and R. S. Oseas. Angiofollicular lymph node hyperplasia (Castle-man's disease) and Kaposi's sarcoma in 2 homosexual males with AIDS, Blood 62 (Suppl. 1):113a (abstract) (1983).
15. R. K. Brynes, W. C. Chan, T. J. Spira et al. Value of lymph node biopsy in unexplained lymphadenopathy in homosexual men, JAMA 250:1313 (1983).
16. H. L. Ioachim, C. W. Lerner and M. L. Tapper. Lymphadenopathies in homosexual men: Relationships with the acquired immune deficiency syndrome, JAMA 250:1306 (1983).
17. C. E. Metroka, S. Cunningham-Rundles, M. S. Pollack et al. Generalized lymphadenopathy in homosexual men, Ann Int Med 99:585 (1983).

18. C. E. Metroka. Generalized lymphadenopathy in homosexual men, in: "AIDS: The Epidemic of Kaposi's Sarcoma and Opportunistic Infections", A. E. Friedman-Kien (with L. J. Laubenstein), ed., Masson, New York (1984).
19. C. Metroka, S. Cunningham-Rundles, J. Mouradian and A. Moore. Generalized lymphadenopathy in intravenous drug users, Blood 62 (Suppl. 1):114a (abstract) (1983).
20. A. E. Pitchenik, M. A. Fischl, G. M. Dickinson et al. Opportunistic infections and Kaposi's sarcoma among Haitians: Evidence of a new acquired immunodeficiency state, Ann Int Med 99:277 (1983).
21. J. E. Menitove, R. H. Aster, J. T. Casper et al. T-lymphocyte subpopulations in patients with classic hemophila treated with cryoprecipitate and lyophilized concentrates, New Engl J Med 308:83 (1983).
22. W. A. Andes, R. D. de Shazo, R. J. Reed, J. C. Harkin and N. Wong. Hemophilic lymphadenopathy: Clinical histologic, cytologic and chromosomal changes in patients with immune deficiency, Blood 62 (Suppl. 1):1082 (abstract) (1983).
23. T. Han, H. Ozer, E. Daday, et al. Clinical and laboratory findings in prison-acquired lymphoproliferative syndrome (PALS) with special reference to AIDS, Blood 62 (Suppl. 1):111a (abstract) (1983).
24. Centers for Disease Control. Immunodeficiency among female sexual partners of males with acquired immune deficiency syndrome (AIDS-New York, Morbid Mortal Weekly Report 31:697 (1983).
25. C. Harris, C. B. Small, R. S. Klein et al. Immunodeficiency in female sexual partners of men with the acquired immunodeficiency syndrome, New Engl J Med 308:1181 (1983).
26. A. J. Pinching, T. J. McManus, D. J. Jeffries et al. Studies of cellular immunity in male homosexuals in London, Lancet ii:126 (1983).
27. J. E. Kaplan, D. B. Fishbein, T. J. Spirz, B. Miller, L. B. Schonberger and P. E. Pinsky. Unexplained generalized lymphadenopathy in homosexual men - the Atlanta experience. This volume.
28. D. I. Abrams. Asymptomatic lymphadenopathy and other early presentations of AIDS, in: "Frontiers of Radiation Therapy and Oncology - Cancer and AIDS", Vol. 19, J. M. Vaeth, ed., Karger Publishing Co., Basal, pp 59-65 (1985).
29. D. Abrams, D. Kiprov, R. Stricker and P. Volberding. Prednisone therapy in AIDS-related immune thrombocytopenia (ITP): Clinical, hematologic and immunologic consequences, Proceedings American Society of Clinical Oncology, Vol. 4 (1985).
30. M. S. Gottlieb, P. R. Wolfe, D. Hardy, A. Jacobs, L. Eppolito, M. G. Sarngadharan, R. C. Gallo and J. L. Fahey. Persistent generalized lymphadenopathy: The UCLA experience. This volume.
31. J. S. Greenspan, D. Greenspan, E. Lennette, M. Conant, D. Abrams, V. Petersen and Y. de Souza. Oral "hairy" leukoplakia - evidence of both papillomavirus & Epstein-Barr virus. This volume.

32. K. L. Moon, M. P. Federle, D. I. Abrams, P. A. Volberding and B. J. Lewis. Kaposi's sarcoma and lymphadenopathy syndrome: Limitations of the abdominal CT in acquired immunodeficiency syndrome, Radiology 150:479 (1984).
33. R. G. Stern, G. Gamsu, J. A. Golden, M. Marji, W. R. Webb and D. I. Abrams. Intrathoracic adenopathy in AIDS and the diffuse, persistent lymphadenopathy syndrome: Diagnostic and clinical implications, Am J Roentgenol 142:689 (1984).
34. U. Mathur-Wagh. Persistent generalized lymphadenopathy in homosexual men. This volume.
35. H. C. Lane, H. Masur, L. C. Egar, et al. Abnormalities of B-cell activation and immunoregulation in patients with the acquired immunodeficiency syndrome, New Engl J Med 309:453 (1983).
36. A. J. Ammann, G. Schiffman, D. I. Abrams, et al. B-cell immunodeficiency in acquired immune deficiency syndrome, JAMA 251:1447 (1984).
37. A. Ammann, D. Abrams, M. Conant, D. Chudwin, M. Cowan, P. A. Volberding, B. Lewis and C. Casavant. Acquired immune dysfunction in homosexual men: Immunologic profiles, Clin Immunol Immunopathol 27:315 (1983).
38. J. A. Golden, D. I. Abrams, R. J. Hattner, et al. Pneumocystis carinii pneumonia in the acquired immunodeficiency syndrome: A diagnostic approach. Submitted.
39. E. De Stefano, R. M. Friedman, A. E. Friedman-Kien, et al. Acid-labile human leukocyte interferon in homosexual men with Kaposi's sarcoma and lymphadenopathy, J Inf Dis 146:451 (1982).
40. K. Welte, N. Ciobanu, G. Kruger et al. Impaired interleukin-2 production in response to PHA and OKT3 antibody in male homosexuals with acquired imune deficiency syndrome: In vitro restoration of T-cell proliferation by highly purified Interleukin-2, in: AIDS: The Epidemic of Kaposi's Sarcoma and Opportunistic Infections, A. E. Friedman-Kien (with L. J. Laubenstein), ed., Masson, New York pp 199-205 (1984).
41. A. R. Moss, G. McCallum, P. A. Volberding, P. Bacchetti, S. Dritz. Mortality associated with mode of presentation in the acquired immune deficiency syndrome, JNCI 73, No. 6:1281 (1984).
42. R. L. Modlin, P. R. Meyer, F. M. Hofman et al. T-lymphocyte subsets in lymph nodes from homosexual men, JAMA 240:1302 (1983).
43. R. W. Enlow, A. Nunez-Roldan, P. Lo Gallo, et al. Increased frequency of HLA-DR5 in lymphadenopathy stage of AIDS. Lancet ii:51 (1983).
44. R. Enlow, D. Mildvan, U. Mathur et al. Acquired immune deficiency syndrome (AIDS): Definition of a prodrome associated with HLA-DR5, Clinical Research 31:342a (1983).
45. M. E. Eyster, J. J. Goedert, P. Man-Chiu, O. T. Preble. Acid-labile alpha interferon. A possible preclinical marker for the acquired immunodeficiency syndrome in hemophilia, New Engl J Med 309:583 (1983).
46. D. I Abrams and P. A. Volberding. Lymphadenopathy in homosexual men: Factors predictive of transformation to AIDS, Proc Am Soc Clin Onc 3:53 (1984).

47. F. Barro-Sinoussi, J. C. Chermann, F. Rey et al. Isolation of a T-lymphotropic retrovirus from a partient at risk for acquired immune deficiency syndrome (AIDS). Science 220:668 (1983).
48. E. P. Gelmann, M. Popovic, D. Blayney et al. Proviral DNA of a retrovirus, human T-cell leukemia virus, in two patients with AIDS. Science 220:862 (1983).
49. R. C. Gallo, P. S. Sarin, E. P. Gelmann et al. Isolation of human T-cell leukemia virus in acquired immunodeficiency syndrome (AIDS), Science 220:865 (1983).
50. B. Poiesz, R. Tomar, S. Merl et al. Detection of human T-cell lymphoma/leukemia virus (HTLV) in patients with acquired immunodeficiency (AIDS) or generalized lymphadenopathy syndrome (GLS), Blood 62 (Suppl. 1):115a (abstract) (1983).

Acknowledgements:

Supported in part by NIH cooperative agreement UOI CA 34980

Special thanks to Nickolin Casciani for assistance with these manuscripts.

THE SYNDROME OF PERSISTENT GENERALIZED LYMPHADENOPATHY: EXPERIENCE WITH 101 PATIENTS

Michael S. Gottlieb, Peter R. Wolfe, John L. Fahey, Steven Knight, David Hardy, Lawrence Eppolito, Ellyn Ashida, Amit Patel, Gildon N. Beall, and Nora Sun

UCLA Center for Health Sciences and Harbor-UCLA Medical Center; Los Angeles, California

There is increasing evidence that infection with the retrovirus LAV/HTLV-III causes a spectrum of outcomes in man ranging from asymptomatic infection to severe immune deficiency complicated by opportunistic infections and neoplasms (1,2). In epidemiologic relationship to the onset of the AIDS epidemic, physicians noted other patients with unexplained fevers, sweats, malaise and in some cases lymphadenopathy (3). These cases were considered related to AIDS in some way, presumably through a common environmental exposure, and the term AIDS-related complex (ARC) was coined by an ad hoc group of intra- and extramural NIH investigators.

The most well-defined, discrete syndrome with features of ARC is the syndrome of persistent generalized lymphadenopathy (PGL), whose appearance has paralleled that of AIDS among population groups known to be at increased risk for AIDS (3-5). The discovery of LAV/HTLV-III shed new light on this syndrome and confirmed widespread clinical suspicions that it was indeed AIDS-related. Published evidence which supports the concept that PGL is one phenotypic outcome of LAV/HTLV-III infection includes i) the ability to culture LAV and HTLV-III from lymph node and peripheral lymphocytes of up to 80 per cent of PGL patients (2), ii) the presence of antibodies to LAV or HTLV-III in 90-100 per cent of these patients (6,7), and iii) observations that a finite number of PGL patients ultimately do develop AIDS as defined by the Centers for Disease Control (3-5).

A single definition of the syndrome of PGL has not yet been accepted by all workers. Most investigators use the following criteria: i) the presence of lymphadenopathy at two or more non-inguinal regions, ii) pdenopathy of 3-6 months duration, and iii) the absence of infections or drug administration known to cause lymphadenopathy (3-5). In some patients lymphadenopathy is associated with constitutional symptoms including malaise, weight loss, diarrhea, fevers and sweats. In other patients lymphadenopathy has been an asymptomatic finding detected on physical examination.

There are no accurate statistics which document the prevalence of PGL, however anecdotal experience in city health clinics suggests that its prevalence in groups at increased risk for AIDS far exceeds the prevalence of the full AIDS syndrome. In this volume Moss and Abrams present information on the prevalence of lymphadenopathy in high-risk San Francisco neighborhoods which confirms this suspicion.

Several clinical research groups have analyzed their experience with PGL. A major aim of these studies has been to determine the risk of progression from PGL to AIDS, and to identify clinical and laboratory features which predict the outcome of the syndrome in the individual patient. A group at the University of California, San Francisco reported that none of 70 patients with PGL followed prospectively developed AIDS over a 12 month period (5). The group at Beth Israel Hospital (New York) observed 7 of 42 patients with PGL progress to AIDS within 12 months (4).

We report here a series of patients with PGL evaluated at the UCLA Center for Health Sciences, and discuss prospects for improved definition and management of this and other syndromes which collectively comprise the AIDS-related complex.

METHODS

Between January, 1982, and December, 1984, approximately 200 patients were evaluated in the Clinical Immunology Clinics of the UCLA Center for the Health Sciences for complaints possibly consistent with ARC. Patients presenting with CDC-defined AIDS were excluded from this series. More than 50% of the ARC patients had had some previous evaluation, and were referred by community physicians. All patients had an extensive interview, medical history, and physical examination at the initial UCLA visit. 101 patients meeting the following criteria for PGL were identified and are the subject of this report. These criteria included: i) lymphadenopathy by examination at 2 or more non-inguinal sites, ii) presence of that lymphadenopathy by history or examination for more than four months, and iii) absence of infection or drug use known to cause lymphadenopathy.

Complete standard laboratory panels were not applied to all patients. In the majority of patients, initial laboratory testing included total white blood cell count, calculated absolute lymphocyte count, red cell indices, quantitative enumeration of T cell subsets, and delayed hypersensitivity skin testing. Antibodies employed for T cell subset testing were Leu 3 (T helper/inducer phenotype) and Leu 2 (T suppressor/cytotoxic phenotype) (8). Skin test antigens included candida, PPD, mumps, and tetanus toxoid. In some cases evaluation included tests for antibody to cytomegalovirus (CMV) and Epstein-Barr virus, VDRL, and *Toxoplasma gondii*.

Lymph node biopsies were processed in paraffin and plastic; samples were cultured and stained for routine organisms and mycobacteria and fungi.

RESULTS

Demographic

The demographic characteristics of our PGL population (Table 1) were similar to those reported in other studies (3-5). Ninety-five percent were homosexual or bisexual. The mean age of all patients was 34 years. The majority of patients had numerous lifetime sexual partners, and all had been sexually active over the three years prior to presentation. Recreational drug use was common, most frequently including marijuana, cocaine and inhalant nitrites (poppers). A past history of sexually-transmitted infections was obtained in 66 per cent; 33 per cent had a history of icteric hepatitis.

Table 1. Characteristics of Study Population (N=101)

Homosexual men:	94%
Intravenous drug users:	8%
Heterosexual men:	5%
Heterosexual women:	1%

Clinical

The mean duration of symptoms prior to the initial UCLA evaluation was 14 months (± 21 SD). The enlarged nodes were frequently asymptomatic, however some patients complained of discomfort associated with fluctuations in lymph node size. Occasional patients with extensive, matted neck nodes had complaints related to lymph node bulk. The patients complaints at presentation are displayed in Table 2.

Table 2. Frequency of Presenting Complaints in Patients with PGL (N=101)

Malaise:	60%
Sweats:	52%
Fevers:	42%
Oral Candida:	32%
Diarrhea:	29%
Zoster:	17%

Forty-three percent had one or more dermatologic complaints, which included seborrhea, generalized skin dryness, impetigo, and cutaneous fungal infections. Two patients had biopsy proven leukocytoclastic angiitis. Twenty-three percent had a past history of herpes zoster. Patients with diarrhea frequently had multiple parasites isolated from their stool, including Entamoeba histolytica, Endolimax nana, Blastocystis hominis, and Entamoeba coli. Many of those with bowel disturbance had a history of previous therapy with metronidazole and diiodoquin, often with minimal improvement.

Abnormalities on physical examination were limited for the most part to the lymphoid, skin and mucous membrane findings. Palpable splenomegaly was present in 11 percent and hepatomegaly in 8 percent. Oral thrush was present in 32 per cent overall.

Immunologic Evaluation

Abnormalities of peripheral blood leukocyte and lymphocyte numbers were common findings. Forty-one percent had leukopenia (less than 4,500 WBC/cubic millimeter). Forty percent were lymphopenic (less than 1,500 lymphocytes/cubic millimeter). At initial evaluation, the mean number of cells/cubic millimeter with the T helper/inducer phenotype (Leu 3) was 293 ± 194 (normal range: 331-1286), and the mean Leu 3/Leu 2 ratio was 0.50 ± 0.35 (normal range: 0.84-2.56).

Serology

Forty of fifty-one patients tested had antibodies to cytomegalovirus present in a titer of at least 1:16. Forty-five of fifty-five patients tested had antibodies to the viral capsid antigen of Epstein-Barr virus (EBV). Tests for antibodies to HTLV-III were applied to serum banked at initial evaluation from 35 patients in this series selected at random. Thirty of these were positive by an enzyme linked immunosorbent assay to whole disrupted HTLV-III using a commercially produced assay under investigation in our laboratory. Western blot analysis of some sera were performed in the laboratory of R. Gallo). Three of the 5 sera which were negative by ELISA were positive for the p24 or p41 antigens or both by the Western blot technique.

The clinical course was of interest in the 2 HTLV-III seronegative patients who met criteria for inclusion in this series. The first seronegative patient presented with lymphadenopathy and a Leu 3/Leu 2 ratio of 0.85 secondary to increased numbers of Leu 2 positive cells. At 13 months following initial evaluation, his lymphadenopathy had resolved and T cell numbers remained stable. CMV antibody was markedly elevated (1:512 by complement fixation). Patient 2 had an illness characterized by lymphadenopathy, a past history of chronic active hepatitis, and recent idiopathic nephrotic syndrome. Leu 3/Leu 2 ratio was initially 0.69 and two years later was 2.17.

Lymph Node Histology

Lymph node biopsies were performed in 16 patients following the first UCLA evaluation. Findings included florid follicular hyperplasia (FH) in 7 patients, and mixed follicular hyperplasia and/or follicular involution with paracortical hyperplasia (mixed pattern) in 9 patients. Patients with the mixed pattern had significant reduction of mean peripheral blood T cell numbers determined with anti-Leu 4 (968/cubic millimeter) compared to patients with FH (2212/cubic millimeter).

Outcome

At least 16/101 patients developed CDC-defined AIDS (7 with Kaposi's sarcoma and 9 with opportunistic infection). Ten died at a mean of 16 months following initial presentation.

For purposes of analysis, the PGL patients were divided into AIDS and non-AIDS groups. The groups were compared with respect to clinical and laboratory parameters present at the initial UCLA evaluation. Between-group comparisons using a corrected chi-square test were performed for the following characteristics: presence of fevers, nightsweats, malaise, weight loss, diarrhea, dermatologic complaints, hepatomegaly, splenomegaly, oral candidiasis, herpes zoster, history of sexually-transmitted disease, history of hepatitis, anergy, lymphopenia, and leukopenia (Tables 3 and 4). The absolute Leu 3 number, and Leu 3/Leu 2 ratio were compared by a two-tailed t test (Table 5). Analyzed as independent variables, the presence at entry of leukopenia, lymphopenia, oral candidiasis, chronic diarrhea and relative paucity of Leu 3-positive lymphocytes predicted the subsequent development of CDC-defined AIDS over the period of observation.

DISCUSSION

Our studies indicate that a subgroup of PGL patients with increased risk of developing AIDS can be identified using several clinical and laboratory parameters. As has been reported by others (4,9), the presence

Table 3. Comparison of frequency of complaints at presentation

Sign/Symptom	Progressed to AIDS	Stable	P value
Diarrhea	88%	23%	0.001
Oral Candida	78%	27%	0.007
Malaise	100%	56%	0.04
Zoster	56%	20%	0.05
Fevers	75%	39%	NS
Weight Loss	67%	35%	NS

Table 4. Comparison of laboratory abnormalities

Finding	Progressed to AIDS	Stable	P value
Anergy	88%	29%	0.004
Leukopenia	88%	36%	0.02
Lymphopenia	88%	42%	0.04

Table 5. Comparison of Leu 3 numbers and Leu 3/Leu 2 ratio at presentation

	Mean Leu 3 cells/ml (± SD)	Leu 3/Leu 2 ratio (± SD)
Progressed	178 ± 145 *	0.30 ± 0.33 **
Stable	314 ± 195 *	0.54 ± 0.34 **

* Difference between groups p=0.024
** Difference between groups p=0.013

of leukopenia, lymphopenia, oral candidiasis, and previous herpes zoster are predictors of an unfavorable outcome. We found that PGL patients developing AIDS had significantly lower T helper/inducer cell numbers compared to patients who had not developed AIDS at the time of the last evaluation. Recent studies in Kaposi's sarcoma indicate similar correlations of T helper cell numbers with survival (J. Fahey, R. Mitsuyasu, manuscript in preparation).

The incidence of progression from PGL to AIDS in our experience (16 per cent) was similar to that reported by Mathur-Wagh. Multiple factors including referral patterns, inclusion criteria and period of follow-up may account for some reported differences in rate of progression. The cumulative incidence of AIDS over a longer period in PGL patients as well as asymptomatic LAV/HTLV-III seropositive individuals is the subject of ongoing assessment.

The definition of the AIDS-related complex (ARC) has been further refined as a result of the several clinical studies of PGL as well as the development of serologic markers for LAV/HTLV-III infection. As originally proposed, the term ARC is too imprecise to be of value for studies of prognosis and therapy. Nevertheless the term served a useful purpose in alerting physicians and public health personnel to the fact that the AIDS epidemic was not limited to cases meeting the CDC surveillance definition. The cumulative evidence is strong that PGL develops in a subgroup of individuals exposed to LAV/HTLV-III. The cofactors which result in chronic lymphadenopathy as a manifestation of the infection and determine progression to AIDS in some cases are incompletely understood and the subject of much current research.

Our studies further indicate that the PGL syndrome is associated in many cases with severe and sometimes progressive T helper lymphopenia and has a very strong association with serologic evidence of LAV/HTLV-III infection. Others have documented a high rate of LAV and HTLV-III isolation from PGL patients (2,5). Our series and others reported in this volume clearly establish that the natural history of PGL is not benign. The cumulative experience with immunotherapy in established AIDS is poor (10). In our view clinical trials of antiviral agents with activity against LAV/HTLV-III, immune response modifiers, and regimens combining these agents are indicated in the PGL syndrome. These trials will permit the assessment safety and efficacy of agents which have potential application in other subgroups of LAV/HTLV-III infected patients.

In hindsight the relationship of some cases previously designated ARC to LAV/HTLV-III infection was doubtful. In our series, two HTLV-III seronegative cases had at least a partial resolution of lymphadenopathy and immunologic abnormality. Serial immunologic studies have remained abnormal in the HTLV-III antibody positive patients. We cannot however completely exclude HTLV-III infection in our two seronegative cases in light of recent findings of HTLV-III isolation from individuals lacking antibody by all detection techniques; however, the symptoms and laboratory findings in these two patients were consistent with diagnoses of other viral infections. Thus our preliminary studies of HTLV-III antibody in PGL indicate that testing for antibody may be of some clinical value in the exclusion of other illnesses associated with lymphadenopathy in patients who are members of AIDS risk groups.

Acknowledgments

Supported by a grant from the National Institutes of Allergy and Infectious Diseases (AI20672) and a grant to the UCLA AIDS Clinical Research Center from the University of California Task Force on AIDS. We thank M. Sarngadharan, P. Markham, and R. Gallo for performing Western-Blot analyses.

References

1. Barre-Sinoussi F, Chermann JC, Rey F, et al. Isolation of a T-lymphotropic virus from a patient at risk for acquired immune deficiency syndrome (AIDS). Science 220:868-71 (1983).

2. Gallo R, Salahuddin S, Popovic M, et al. Frequent detection and isolation of cytopathic retroviruses (HTLV-III) from patients with AIDS and at risk for AIDS. Science 224:500-03 (1984).
3. Metroka CE, Cunningham-Rundles S, Pollack MS, et al. Generalized lymphadenopathy in homosexual men. Ann Int Med. 99:585-91 (1983).
4. Mathur-Wagh U, Enlow RW, Spigland I, et al. Longitudinal study of persistent generalized lymphadenopathy in homosexual men: relation to the acquired immune deficiency syndrome. Lancet i:1033-8 (1984).
5. Abrams DI, Lewis BJ, Beckstead JH, et al. Persistent diffuse lymphadenopathy in homosexual men: endpoint or prodrome? Ann Int Med. 100:801-8 (1984).
6. Safai B, Sarngadharan MG, Groopman JE, et al. Seroepidemiologic studies of HTLV-III in AIDS. Lancet i:1438-40 (1984).
7. Brun-Vezinet F, Barre-Sinoussi F, Saimot AG, et al. Detection of IgG antibodies to lymphadenopathy-associated virus in patients with AIDS or lymphadenopathy syndrome. Lancet i:1253-6 (1984).
8. Schroff RS, Gottlieb MS, Prince HE, et al. Immunologic studies of homosexual men with immunodeficiency and Kaposi's sarcoma. Clin. Immunol. and Immunopathol. 27:300-14 (1983).
9. Klein RS, Harris CA, Small CB, et al. Oral candidiasis in high risk patients as the initial manifestation of the acquired immune deficiency syndrome. N Engl J Med. 311:354-58 (1984).
10. Gottlieb MS, Wolfe PR, Mitsuyasu RT. Immunotherapy of the acquired immune deficiency syndrome. In: Advances in Host Defense Mechanisms, Gallin J and Fauci A, (eds.) New York: Raven Press (1985).

LONGITUDINAL ASSESSMENT OF PERSISTENT GENERALIZED LYMPHADENOPATHY (PGL) IN HOMOSEXUAL MEN

Usha Mathur-Wagh[1], Donna Mildvan[1], Ilya Spigland[2], Francoise Brun-Vezinet[3], Francoise Barre-Sinoussi[4], Luc Montagnier[4], and Jean Claude Chermann[4]

[1]The Department of Medicine, Beth Israel Medical Center; The Mount Sinai School of Medicine of the City University of New York, New York
[2]Division of Virology, Montefiore Hospital and Medical Center; Albert Einstein College of Medicine, Bronx, New York
[3]Laboratoire de Virologie, Hôpital Claude Bernard Paris, France
[4]Unite d'Oncologie Virale, Institut Pasteur, 24 Rue du Docteur Roux, 75015 Paris, France

Since February, 1981, a cohort of 42 homosexual or bisexual men with persistent generalized lymphadenopathy (PGL) has been followed longitudinally at the Beth Israel Medical Center (BIMC), with periodic clinical, virologic and immunologic evaluations. We defined the syndrome of PGL in homosexual and bisexual men (1,2) by the presence of: a) lymph nodes of greater than 1 cm size, of more than 3 months duration, involving at least 2 extrainguinal anotomic sites; b) absence of symptomatic infection at the onset of lymphadenopathy; c) absence of an apparent etiology such as history of intravenous drug abuse, dilantin therapy, recent immunization, skin rash or evidence of neoplastic disease, and d) absence of unexplained weight loss, diarrhea, thrush or evidence of other opportunistic infections or cancers. A detailed description of the epidemiologic, clinical and laboratory findings of this group has been previously reported (3).

Outcome: During the initial 18 months of prospective evaluation, 6 of 42 patients (14%) progressed to AIDS (5 with Kaposi's sarcoma (KS), 1 with non-Hodgkin's lymphoma) (1). After 30 months, with the development of AIDS in 2 additional patients (1 with Pneumocystis carinii pneumonia (PCP) and 1 with simultaneous KS and PCP), the complication rate was 19% (3). At the most recent follow-up of 40 months, 2 additional patients developed AIDS. One patient was found to have KS and the other PCP, bringing the current progression rate to 24% (10/42).

The mean duration of lymphadenopathy prior to the diagnosis of AIDS was 24 months. However, the duration of lymphadenopathy in patients who developed either PCP (mean 39 months) or non-Hodgkin's lymphoma (mean 42 months) was longer, when compared to patients who developed KS (mean 16 months) (Table 1).

Table 1. DURATION OF LYMPHADENOPATHY PRIOR TO DIAGNOSIS

Diagnosis (n)	Mean Duration in Months (range)
Kaposi's sarcoma (KS) (6)	16 (4 - 30)
Pneumocystis carinii pneumonia (PCP) (2)	39 (36 - 42)
Non Hodgkin's lymphoma (1)	42 (-)
KS & PCP (1)	22 (-)

A change in lymph node size was helpful in predicting outcome in the 10 patients who developed AIDS. Four of the 7 patients who developed either KS or non-Hodgkin's lymphoma showed a 3 fold increase in lymph node size, whereas 3 of 3 patients who developed PCP either alone or in combination with KS, had a 3 fold decrease in lymph node size prior to diagnosis. A similar reduction in lymph node size was also noted in 10 of the remaining 32 patients who have not yet developed AIDS. Whether an improvement in lymph node size in these individuals represents a sign of recovery or early occult AIDS, remains to be seen.

Serological Studies: IgG antibodies to LAV (lymphadenopathy associated virus) were determined using an ELISA technique, the details of which have been described elsewhere (4). Briefly, this assay was performed with a purified and disruped LAV preparation. A lysate of uninfected lymphocytes was used as a control antigen. Each serum was tested (1:40 dilution) in duplicate against both viral and control antigens. Sera were considered positive when differential optical density was more than 0.30. On each plate, a positive control serum was tested at 4 dilutions, and a standard curve was used to measure the height of the antibody titer. A titer of 1:40 or greater was considered positive.

LAV antibody titers were performed on 38 of 42 PGL patients, 24 patients with documented AIDS (including 3 patients who progressed from PGL to AIDS), and 12 hospital worker controls (Table 2). Seventy-six percent of patients with PGL and 71% of patients with AIDS had detectable antibody. Although the prevalance of antibody in our patients is similar to that described by others (4,5), higher rates of seropositivity using a combination of ELISA and western blot techniques have been reported recently (6). The 12 hospital personnel were chosen for LAV antibody studies on the basis of their frequent and close contact with AIDS patients and specimens in the preceding 2 years. None of these individuals were found to be seropositive. This information together with the observation that AIDS has not spread significantly to populations outside the original high risk groups, further suggests that transmission of infection through casual contact is unlikely.

LAV antibody status of the 32 PGL patients in the cohort who thus far have not developed AIDS is presented in Table 3. Testing was performed on paired sera obtained at a mean interval of 14 months. Twenty-five patients were seropositive and 7 were seronegative. Among the 25 seropositive patients, 4 had a four fold decrease in titer, 2 of which became seronegative. Three had a four fold increase in titer and in the remaining 18 patients LAV titers remained unchanged. There was no difference in the various historical, clinical or laboratory parameters in the seronegative patients when compared to those of the seropositive patients. The implications of a four fold rise or a fall in LAV titers and a change from seropositive to seronegative state as observed in 2 of our patients are unclear at the present time.

Conclusions: 1) PGL progresses to CDC defined AIDS in a significant proportion (24%) of patients followed longitudinally for up to 40 months. Kaposi's sarcoma appears earlier following PGL than either PCP or non-Hodgkin's lymphoma; 2) a change in the lymph node size may serve as a clue to the ultimate AIDS diagnosis; patients with KS usually present with a significant increase and those with PCP with a significant decrease in lymph node size prior to diagnosis; and 3) the demonstration of a high prevalance of antibody to LAV in this original cohort of PGL patients collected as early as 1981, adds to the accumulating evidence that implicates LAV as the cause of PGL and AIDS.

Table 2. SERUM IgG, ELISA ANTIBODY TITERS TO LAV

Diagnosis (n)	No. Positive (%)	Mean Antibody (range)
PGL (38)	29 (76%)	1:304 (1:40 - 1:1600)
AIDS (24)	17 (71%)	1:203 (1:40 - 1:1600)
Hospital Worker Controls (12)	0	0

Table 3. LAV IgG ELISA IN PGL PATIENTS WHO HAVE NOT DEVELOPED AIDS

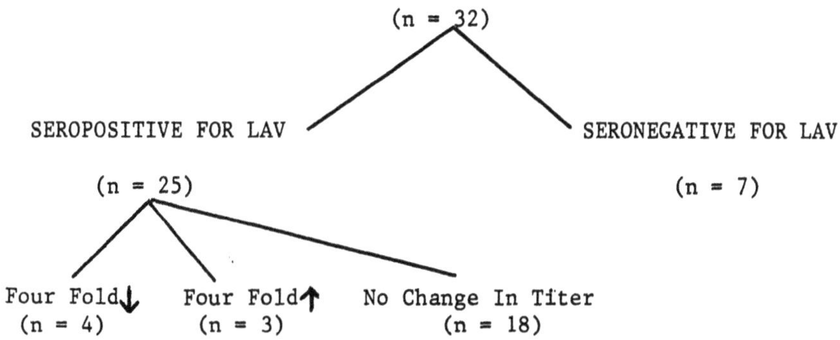

REFERENCES

1. Mildvan D, Mathur U, Enlow RW, et al. Persistent generalized lymphadenopathy among homosexual males. CDC: Morbid. Mortal. Wkly. Rep. 1982; 31:249-251.

2. Mathur U*, Enlow RW, Spigland I, William DC, Winchester RJ, Mildvan D. Generalized lymphadenopathy: A prodrome of Kaposi's sarcoma in male homosexuals? *Abstract presented at the 22nd Interscience Conference on Antimicrobial Agents and chemotherapy, Miami Beach, Florida, October 1982.

3. Mathur-Wagh U, Enlow RW, Spigland I, et al. Longitudinal study of persistent generalized lymphadenopathy (PGL) in homosexual men: relationship to the acquired immune deficiency syndrome. Lancet 1984; 1033-38.

4. Brun-Vezinet F, Rouzioux C, Barre-Sinoussi F, et al. Detection of IgG antibodies to lymphadenopathy assoicated virus in patients with AIDS or lymphadenopathy syndrome. Lancet 1984; 1253-56.

5. Sarngadharan MG, Popovic M, Bruch L, Schupbach J, Gallo RC. Antibodies reactive with human T-lymphotropic retroviruses (HTLV-III) in the serum of patients with AIDS. Science 1984; 224:506-8.

6. Safai B, Sarngadharan MG, Groopman JE, et al. Seroepidemiological studies of human T-lymphotropic retroviruses type III in acquired immune deficiency syndrome. Lancet 1984, 1:1438-40.

CYTOTOXIC EFFECTOR MECHANISMS IN AIDS

S. Cunningham-Rundles, C.E. Metroka, B. Safai, M. Krim,
B.Y. Rubin and G. Hayward

Memorial Sloan-Kettering Cancer Center
1275 York Avenue
New York, NY

INTRODUCTION

The development of the Acquired Immunodeficiency Disease Syndrome, AIDS, in the United States has occurred primarily in certain groups, i.e. homosexual and bisexual men (1,2), I.V. drug abusers (3,4), Haitians (5), and hemophiliacs receiving Factor VIII concentrates (6). Evidence for AIDS in blood transfusion recipients and children of drug abusing or Haitian parents associated with apparent transmission of a newly described retrovirus, HTLV-III, LAV (7,8) has provoked study of critical conditions for AIDS development. It seems logical to assume that AIDS develops in a series of stages, the earliest of which may not be accompanied by any obvious clinical symptoms. Deficiencies in cell mediated immunity have been clearly documented by ourselves and others in patients with AIDS-related opportunistic infections (9,10) and AIDS-related Kaposi's sarcoma. In addition, we and others have focused much attention upon homosexual men with generalized lymphadenopathy (11-14). Although these patients do not fit the criteria for CDC defined AIDS at the present time, we have observed that an increasingly large number of our originally described population have gone on to develop CDC defined AIDS (11).

Present evidence supports the view that a retrovirus infecting the T helper lymphocyte subpopulation is a critical factor in the initiation of a prodrome state. At present, it is not known whether this prodrome can be resolved by natural host defense mechanisms in an individual with an intact immune system. This is partly because all of the identified risk groups appear to have moderate to severe immunocompromise as a consequence of life style factors, including drug abuse, unusual exposure to potentially pathogenic agents, immaturity of the immune system (children), exposure to foreign antigens (including allogeneic cells in homosexuals, hemophiliacs, transfusion recipients). Possible significance of genetic factors has also been suggested. We have been interested in tracing the development of immune deficiency which we hypothesized might have begun as an increasingly deregulated response (10) to antigenic stimulation. In light of present understanding, it is reasonable to suggest that the presence of the retrovirus may serve to alter immunoregulation so that recognition and response do not occur normally. In the work presented here, we have endeavored to study alteration in cytotoxic mechanisms that might accompany central deregulation in AIDS. For this purpose we have focused our studies on analysis of endogenous, interferon augmented, and activated natural killer (NK) activity in AIDS patients, patients with generalized lymphadenopathy at risk for AIDS (AIDS-LA), AIDS associated Kaposi's sarcoma (AIDS-KS), and AIDS associated opportunistic infection (AIDS-OI), use of AIDS patients' and AIDS-LA fresh peripheral blood mononuclear cells (PBM) as targets of cytotoxicity by normal effector cytotoxic cells, and studies of cell lines spontaneously established from AIDS patients as targets of cytolytic destruction by effector cells from AIDS patients' PBM and normal controls.

The purpose of the first approach was to delineate and characterize the functional capacity of the NK system in AIDS patients against a universally recognized, NK sensitive tumor target. The goal of the second approach was to determine whether or not possible alterations in the T cell surface might render AIDS patients' cells sensitive to NK lysis since it is known that normal thymocytes (expressing tumor-associated antigens) can be recognized and destroyed by normal nonsensitized effector cells (15). The aim of the third approach was to define the cell type of spontaneously outgrown cells and to determine the nature and possible restriction of cytotoxic effector mechanisms directed toward such cells using homogeneous populations of cells.

MATERIALS AND METHODS

Cell Preparation

Peripheral blood mononuclear cells were isolated from venous blood by density gradient centrifugation technique, washed three times in Hank's Balanced Salt Solution (HBSS, Grand Island Biological Company, Grand Island, NY) and resuspended in RPMI 1640 (Gibco) containing glutamine (0.23 mg/ml), penicillin (10 I.U./ml), streptomycin (10 μg/ml), and 10% pooled normal human serum (PNHS) as described previously (16). Lymph node cells were obtained from fresh lymph node biopsy material and prepared by teasing with 18-gauge sterile needles followed by 2 washes in HBSS prior to resuspension in RPMI 1640 as described above.

Establishment of Cell Lines

Cell lines were established from patients with generalized lymphadenopathy at risk for AIDS by isolating peripheral blood mononuclear cells and culturing at several densities (2×10^6 to 0.5×10^6 lymphocytes/ml) in one ml cultures in 24-well Linbro flat-bottomed plates in RPMI 1640 supplemented with 15% heat in activated fetal calf serum (Microbiological Associates, Walkenville, MD). Cell lines became established after 5 to 6 weeks and were expanded in T-25 flasks in larger volumes as required for the studies described.

Patient Populations

Patient groups have been previously described (11) and consisted of patients with generalized lymphadenopathy at risk for AIDS with no identified underlying cause for either lymphadenopathy or immune deficiency and no relevant medical history and patients who fit the CDC surveillance criteria for AIDS. In some cases patients subsequently developed AIDS and these instances are identified in the text.

Controls for these studies were employees at MSKCC with no known risk factors for AIDS.

Cytotoxicity Assays

Cytotoxicity was studied using either freshly isolated effector cells or 'activated' effector cells against either the K562 erythroleukemia target, freshly isolated peripheral blood mononuclear cells or established cell lines. The K562 tumor cell line has been continuously maintained in suspension culture. The cell lines from lymphadenopathy patients grew as semi-detached cultures and were removed by pipetting.

Putative target and control target cells were labelled with 0.25 mCi/ 2×10^6 cells Chromium^{51} (New England Nuclear Corporation, Boston, MA) for 1 hour, washed, and plated at 1×10^4 targets/well. Incubation with effector cells was carried out at a range of effector:target ratios (100:1 to 10:1) in different experiments. Each effector:target ratio was prepared in triplicate for each ratio tested in round-bottomed microtiter plates (Vangaard, Neptune, NJ) and incubated for 4 hours at 37^0C in a humid incubator containing 5% CO_2. Target cells were plated alone to obtain spontaneous release, and target cells with Triton X-100 were plated to obtain total release. Incubation period for studies with K562 was 4 hours; incubation period for AIDS cell lines was 18 hours. Following incubation and centrifugation, aliquots of the supernatants were counted in a gamma scintillation counter and data were quantified according to the formula:

$$\% \text{ experimental release} = \frac{(\text{experimental release} - \text{spontaneous release})}{(\text{total release} - \text{spontaneous release})}$$

Method follows that previously published (17).

Activation of Cytotoxicity

Cytotoxicity was induced in experiments conducted as described above within the assay period using interferon-alpha (r-IFN-Aα). IFN α was obtained from Hoffman-LaRoche, Nutley, NJ through the courtesy of Dr. S.E. Krown and Dr. H.F. Oettgen. 800 U were added at multiple concentrations of effector cells. Cytotoxicity was also induced using a 6-day culture period with 5-8 $\times 10^6$ mononuclear cells/flask, or lymph node (LN) cells. Activators were r-IFN-Aα, *E. coli* prepared as described previously (16), and Orthoclone, OKT-3 (obtained as a gift from Dr. G. Goldstein, Ortho Pharmaceuticals, Raritan, NJ). Method follows that previously published (18).

Interferon Measurement

Interferon activity was measured as inhibition of the cytopathic effect produced by vesicular stomatitis virus (VSV) on GM2767 (human fibroblasts trisomic for chromosome G-21) or Marin Darby Bovine Kidney (MDBK) cells. Culture supernatants were analyzed following the activation period. Data presented using IFN α to activate natural killer (NK) cells are given with starting concentration of IFN α netted out.

Hybridization Analysis

Cell samples were studied by one of us (G.H.) for evidence of Epstein Barr virus (EBV) and cytomegalovirus (CMV). The methods were DNA by dot blot and Southern blot hybridization using cloned viral DNA fragment sources at Johns Hopkins Medical Center as previously described (19).

Cell Surface Marker Analysis

Cell surface markers were determined using flow cytometric analysis of stained cells with monoclonal T cell markers including OKT-3, OKT-4, OKT-8, OKT-11 (Orthoclone), and B-1, B-2 (Coulter).

Antibodies to HTLV-III

Assessment of antibodies to HTLV-III was conducted by Dr. Richard M. Thorn (Cambridge BioScience) using immunofluorescence technique with HTLV-III positive and negative standard cell lines.

RESULTS

Natural Killer (NK) Activity

Natural killer activity against the erythroleukemia tumor cell line, K562, was studied with cells derived from peripheral blood of patients with generalized lymphadenopathy at risk for AIDS (AIDS-LA) and untreated patients with AIDS associated Kaposi's sarcoma (AIDS-KS). The patients had been followed over the course of 2 to 3 years and the following observations may be briefly described:

Among patients with AIDS-LA, 22 of 35, or 62%, had less than 14.7% endogenous cytotoxicity toward the K562 target at an effector:target ratio of 100:1, which was the ratio giving maximal lysis of the target. This was below the lowest normal response previously observed in this system in age- and sex-matched normal controls (17). Results obtained with repeated testing of these patients suggested that three subgroups could be defined: 1) Low Activity: 23% of AIDS-LA patients showed activity less than 6% with a range of 0% to 5%. 2) Midrange Activity: 63% of AIDS-LA patients had activity in the range of 9% to 21%. 3) High Activity: 14% of AIDS-LA patients had activity in the range of 29% to 57%. Individual patients with initially 'high activity' showed a sharp decline in level of endogenous cytotoxicity prior to the development of AIDS as defined by the CDC.

Among patients with AIDS-KS, 7 of 21, of 33%, had abnormal NK activity toward K562. No clustering of patients into different levels of cytotoxic activity could be demonstrated. Those with the lowest level of spontaneous NK activity (less than 12%) developed opportunistic infections and showed immediate disease progression.

Examination of endogenous NK activity in 5 patients with classical KS (non-AIDS) indicated decreased NK function in 3 of 5 as shown in Table 1 (Cases 2 and 4):

Table 1. Endogenous NK Activity in Classical AIDS

Case	% Cytotoxicity at E:T ratio 100:1	50:1	25:1
1	41.2	27.5	16.4
2	0.5	0.4	0.0
3	23.0	20.7	17.5
4	11.2	8.7	7.7
5	10.9	6.9	3.4

These results indicate that decreased NK function in AIDS-KS cannot be strictly attributable to AIDS. Augmentation of anti-K562 activity was undertaken using IFN α to rec ruit pre NK cells. Studies on patients with AIDS-LA in the short-term ^{51}Cr release assay showed that in 50% of cases peripheral blood mononuclear cell NK activity could not be augmented. One half of those patients with normal or high endogenous cytotoxic activity could also not be boosted <u>in vitro</u>. Among patients with AIDS_KS, 40% were found to have virtual depletion of precursor NK cells as measured by lack of augmentation with IFN α, and 50% with endogenous activity within normal range could not be augmented.

'Activated' Cytotoxicity Toward K562 in AIDS

The observed absence of inducible NK activity within the short-term ^{51}Cr release assay in patients with AIDS-KS and AIDS-LA who had levels of endogenous NK activity within the normal range suggested that depletion of precursor NK cells might have occurred. However, it also seemed possible that NK function might have been down-regulated or suppressed *in vivo*. A more rigorous study of this was undertaken by stimulating PBM during a 6-day culture period with IFN α, IFN γ, *E. coli*, an IFN γ inducer, and OKT-3, an IFN γ inducer. Data are shown in Table 2:

Table 2. Activated and Endogenous Natural Killer Activity in AIDS and Patients with AIDS-LA

	Percent Lysis					
Diagnosis	Endogenous	Activated in 6-Day Culture Activator				
	(Fresh)	none	IFNα[2]	IFNγ	E. coli[3]	OKT3
1. LA	22.1	13.6	63.2	47.0	59.4	15.0
2. LA[1]	21.1	27.0	47.7	67.5	67.5	48.3
3. KS	15.3	7.6	17.5	29.3	18.8	32.4
4. LA	16.5	19.6	30.4	33.6	41.7	13.2
5. LA	28.8	23.3	40.7	43.5	62.8	16.5
6. KS	3.8	16.0	14.5	31.4	5.5	49.9
7. LA	20.4	35.5	67.1	64.1	65.0	48.5
8. LA	3.5	4.2	30.8	50.2	49.7	9.7
9. LA[1]	3.2	2.2	0.4	10.2	10.1	ND
10. LA	12.8	13.8	26.8	39.5	14.3	24.4

[1] Subsequently developed AIDS

[2] Normal control - 6 days - IFN α induced NK:
range: 32.1 - 62.3 %
median: 45.9 %

[3] Normal control - 6 days - IFN γ induced NK:
range: 35.5 - 83.2 %
median: 64.2 %

In two instances, Cases 6 and 7, increase in endogenous activity was seen in absence of any *in vitro* activator (cultures were not stimulated with fetal calf serum). In 7 of 10 instances IFN α augmented NK activity, and in 9 of 10 instances IFN γ activation was associated with significant increase in cytotoxic activity. In one instance, case 9, increase to a low level of function was observed. Marked augmentation was seen in 8 of 10 studies when *E. coli* was used to activate cytotoxicity and in 5 of 10 instances when OKT-3 was utilized. Expression of cytotoxicity after 6 days was accompanied by secretion of IFN α or γ into the culture supernatant. Data shown in Table 3 demonstrate that *E. coli* and OKT-3 induced production of IFN γ that was not always associated with the expression of cytotoxicity as shown in the first case (lines 1-4). Similarly, IFN α induction led to further IFN α secretion (Data in Table 3 show net production of IFN α with initial added IFN α netted out) that was not always accompanied by cytotoxicity (see line 2). Presumably a higher level of cytotoxicity might have been present at an earlier stage of culture.

Peripheral Blood Mononuclear Cells from AIDS Patients as Targets for Cytotoxicity

The observation that endogenous NK activity was high in some patients with AIDS-related lymphadenopathy suggested that *in vivo* activation might have occurred. We also observed 'spontaneous' activation of peripheral blood mononuclear cells, PBM, as reflected by incorporation of ^{14}C thymidine in the absence of activation *in vitro* (data not shown). In some patients spontaneous lymphocyte proliferation was accompanied by interferon secretion *in vitro* as previously described by us (20). Although fresh peripheral blood mononuclear cells cannot be killed as targets of unprimed cytotoxicity, it seemed possible that lymphocytes from AIDS patients might, if new antigens associated with transformation or differentiation antigens were expressed. Therefore, PBM from AIDS-OI and AIDS-KS patients were labelled with ^{51}Cr and used as targets with freshly isolated effector cells from healthy volunteers in an 18-hour cytotoxicity assay. As shown in Figure 1, in 4 of 9 cases, cytotoxicity against the AIDS-KS or AIDS-OI PBM could be demonstrated.

Table 3. Correlation Between NK Activity and Interferon Production

Diagnosis		Cell Source	Culture Addition	% Cytotoxicity 100:1	50:1	Interferon Generated[1]
1.	KS	PBL	none	16.0	11.7	0
2.	"	"	IFNα[2]	14.5	7.5	200
3.	"	"	E.coli[3]	5.5	3.9	30
4.	"	"	OKT3	49.9	39.1	60
5.	LA	PBL	none	35.5	27.0	0
6.	"	"	IFNα	67.1	6.0	100
7.	"	"	E.coli	65.0	48.5	600
8.	"	"	OKT3	48.5	40.3	20
9.	LA	LN	none	8.4	4.7	0
10.	"	"	IFNα	48.1	40.3	1200
11.	"	"	E.coli	61.9	61.4	20

[1] Units/ml culture supernatant

[2] Interferon α produced = final concentration - original addition

[3] Interferon γ produced by *E. coli* and OKT3 stimulated cultures

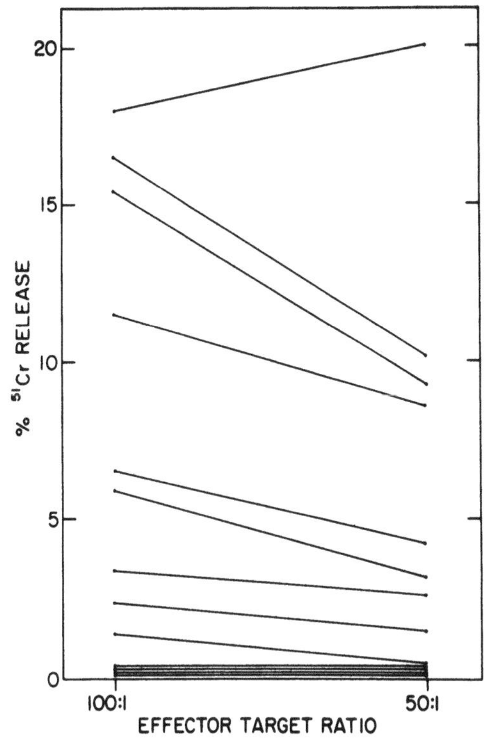

Figure 1. Cytotoxicity of Normal Effector Cells Expressed Against PBM from AIDS-OI and AIDS-KS

Table 4. Relationship Between ^{51}Chromium Binding and Susceptibility to Lysis

Target Source	Spontaneous Release	Total Release	Experimental Release[1]
Fresh Normal PBL	178	508	0
Fresh AIDS PBL-1	294	2032	15.4
Fresh AIDS PBL-2	196	1868	16.5
Fresh AIDS PBL-3	180	490	0
Fresh AIDS PBL-4	269	2004	11.5
Fresh AIDS PBL-5	301	1986	3.4
Fresh AIDS PBL-6	196	1942	5.9
Fresh AIDS PBL-7	236	1386	1.4
Fresh AIDS PBL-8	164	908	6.5
Fresh AIDS PBL-9	416	3488	18.0

[1] Percent Lysis

As shown in Table 4, there was no correlation between the ability of the AIDS PBM to take up ^{51}Cr or to undergo spontaneous lysis and the level of cytotoxicity observed.

In subsequent experiments, it was determined that patients with AIDS-LA and no constitutional symptoms did not have PBM that could serve as targets for cytotoxicity by unprimed effector cells from normal persons. In addition patients with advanced AIDS or patients with AIDS-KS on IFN treatment did not have PBM susceptible to cytotoxic lysis.

Spontaneously established cell lines were grown from unseparated PBM from patients with AIDS-LA. These cell lines could be established without Interleukin-2, IL-2, supplementation, and once established in regular growth medium did not show a tendency to spontaneous regression. The cell lines were found to contain multiple copies of the EBV genome by DNA hybridization analysis. The cell lines were found to secrete moderate to large amounts of acid labile IFN .

Flow cytometry was used to determine cell surface markers. The lines discussed in the present paper did not express T cell markers, but about 20% to 30% of the cells expressed certain B cell markers (Coulter B-1, B-2).

These presumed B cell lines containing multiple EBV genomes were not lysed by freshly isolated normal effector cells from 9 volunteers (0 to 1% cytotoxicity). However, some cytotoxicity toward the cell lines was seen when IFN α was added (1% to 10%) with 6 of the effector cells showing lysis in the range of 5% to 10%. In contrast, 5 of 11 AIDS patients had endogenous cytotoxic activity toward an AIDS cell line target in the range 5% to 20%, and 3 additional patients showed slight ability to lyse the target. Following incubation with IFN α, 9 of 11 AIDS patients were able to lyse this target with resulting percent killing ranging from 8% to 33%. Six patients lysed more than 15% of the targets. The studies reported above were carried out using a single reference AIDS-LA cell line as target. The patient from whom this cell line was started had antibodies to HTLV-III. Other cell lines used as targets are shown in Figure 2, where two different AIDS cell lines were used as targets for a single AIDS-LA patient's effector cells. As shown, the addition of IFN α led to significant augmentation of cytotoxicity.

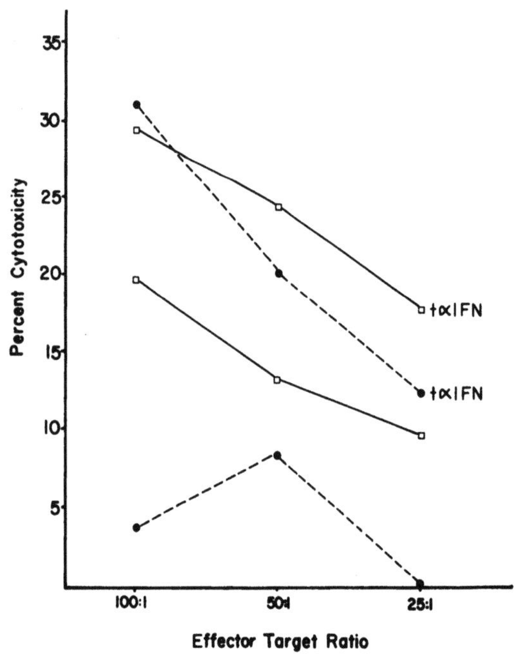

Figure 2. Lysis of Two AIDS Cell Lines by AIDS Patient Effector Cells

The next series of experiments were aimed at determining whether or not an AIDS patient's effector cells would preferentially lyse autologous LCL cells. Data are shown in Figure 3.

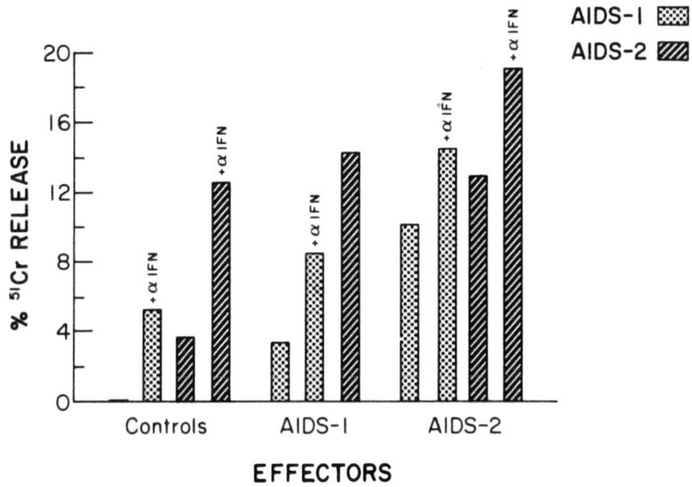

Figure 3. Lysis of AIDS-LCL by Autologous and Allogeneic AIDS-LA Effector Cells

As shown, lysis by normal control effector PBM of the AIDS-LA-1 target occurred only in the presence of IFN α, and lysis of the AIDS-LA-2 target was significant only in the presence of IFN α. The AIDS-LA-1 effector cell showed little autologous lysis of the AIDS-LA-1 target and showed augmentation with IFN α. Lysis of the allogeneic target, AIDS-LA-2, was greater. The AIDS-LA-2 effector cell showed ability to lyse both the allogeneic and the autologous targets, and IFN α had a moderately augmenting effect.

In an effort to determine whether or not there might be cross recognition of target structures expressed on AIDS-LCL and K562 cell lines, effector cells were incubated with a fixed concentration of labelled K562 (hot) and increasing concentrations of unlabelled (cold) AIDS-LCL target cells. Endogenous lysis of the targets alone at different effector:target ratios is shown in the table below:

Table 5a. Relative Lysis of K562 and AIDS-LCL Cytotoxicity Toward K562

Case	Diagnosis	Effector:Target Ratio 100:1	50:1	25:1
A	Control	89.7	85.4	79.9
B	AIDS-KS	25.2	25.1	19.7
C	AIDS-KS	71.0	64.8	50.2
D	Classical AIDS	66.2	65.5	56.9

Table 5b. Cytotoxicity Toward AIDS-1

Case	Diagnosis	Effector:Target Ratio 100:1	50:1	25:1
A	Control	4.7	6.3	2.2
B	AIDS-KS	4.6	1.0	0.0
C	AIDS-KS	31.1	17.8	7.2
D	Classical AIDS	0	0	0

As shown in Study C, only the AIDS-KS effector cell was able to lyse the AIDS-1 LCL. As shown in Figure 4, cold K562 target cells were effective in reducing measured lysis of the hot K562 target for all effector cells, but AIDS-1 LCL did not compete against K562.

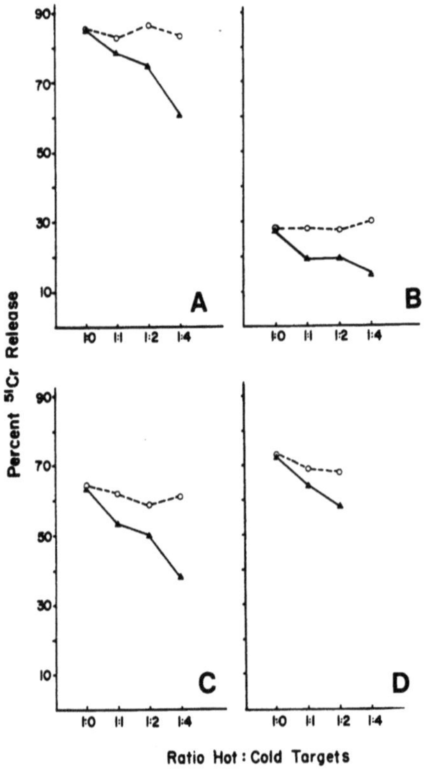

KEY: ▶-▶-▶ K562
0-0-0 AIDS-1 LCL

Figure 4. Cold Target Inhibition of K562 Cytotoxicity (For identity of effector cells, see Table 5)

DISCUSSION

The data presented here demonstrate that depressed NK activity is a feature of AIDS and can be observed in patients with generalized lymphadenopathy associated with risk of AIDS, AIDS-LA. Endogenous NK activity was frequently found in the absence of inducibility by NK augmenting agents, demonstrating that depletion of the precursor compartment could occur independently of the mature NK compartment. Alternatively, this observation could reflect deregulatory or functional inactivation of precursor NK cells. We have recently found that elevated acid labile IFN α is sera of AIDS-LA patients is a pre-clinical marker with prognostic value for predicting the development of CDC defined AIDS within a 3 to 21 month period (C. Metroka, et al., in press). Earlier findings suggested that spontaneous restoration of NK function might accompany a regenerating immune system in AIDS-LA (20). The interferon system has been implicated in self regulation of the NK system (21). In patients with AIDS-OI, Lopez et al. (22) have reported absence of interferon α induction <u>in vitro</u>. Similarly, Murray et al. (23) have demonstrated absence of interferon γ production in patients with AIDS. Recently Levin et al. (24) have demonstrated hyperactivation of the interferon system in vitro among healthy homosexuals at risk for AIDS. We and others have found that a subset of healthy homosexuals at risk for AIDS have hyperactivity of the NK system and may have cellular populations that spontaneously secrete interferon and mediate strong cytotoxicity toward NK sensitive targets when T cells were stimulated by autologous B cells in the autologous mixed lymphocyte culture reaction.

Melder and Ho (25) have shown that administration of interferon inducers in vivo produces hyper-response of the NK system followed by hypo-response in which induction in vitro is also abolished. The phenomenon of the development of NK refractoriness to induction by interferon in vitro has also been described in patients receiving interferon therapy by Golub et al. (26). We have found that acid labile IFN α from AIDS patients is an excellent inducer of NK activity using normal PBM. These findings as a whole support the concept that interferons are induced in response to antigenic or other stimulation in AIDS and that hyper-reactivity precedes the evolution and expression of the hypo-responsiveness that characterizes CDC defined AIDS.

The incidence of EBV virus in AIDS patients has been found by ourselves and others to be essentially 100%. Although the possible role of this virus in the etiology of AIDS has not been clarified, we and others have observed a strikingly increased incidence of B cell lymphomas in AIDS patients (11-13). In the present paper we report that cell lines that can be established from PBL of AIDS patients have B cell characteristics, contain multiple copies of the EBV genome, and secrete large amounts of IFN α, much or all of which is acid labile (manuscript in preparation). The lines discussed in this report were made from AIDS-LA patients with antibodies to HTLV-III. Since Purtillo et al. (these preceedings) have demonstrated presence of HTLV-III in B cells from AIDS patients, it is reasonable to assume that B cells carrying retrovirus and EBV could and would be recognized in the development of immune response in AIDS.

EBV is a B-lymphotropic herpes virus that acts as a polyclonal B cell activator, stimulating cell division with the generation of continuous B cell lines in vitro. In EBV-induced infectious mononucleosis, this activation is usually followed by extensive proliferation of immunoregulatory T cells, which appear in blood as atypical lymphocytes with expression of IA antigen as a sign of activation and a surface phenotype comparable to mature thymocytes as shown by reactivity with the monoclonal antibody OKT-10 (27). Cells bearing this phenotype have been seen in AIDS patients (1) and may have been the target bearing cells in our observed normal effector cell cytotoxicity directed against AIDS patients' PBM reported here, since thymocytes have been shown to serve as NK targets (15). Virus specific T cell memory has been found to accompany the normal course of infectious mononucleosis so that culture of PBM from such donors regresses spontaneously owing to the presence of cytotoxic T cells (28). Since we established our cell lines from seropositive donors, using unseparated PBM, and did not observe regression of outgrowth, we conclude that normal regulation has been abrogated. This deregulation could occur at different levels, affecting development and expression of cytotoxic cells or susceptibility of the target to lysis so that within 5 to 6 weeks the cell population has B cell characteristics. Attempts to establish T cell lines spontaneously have been ineffective.

CTL activated in vivo during primary response to EBV have been found to lyse autologous targets preferentially; the possibility of HLA restriction has been suggested (30). NK activity has been found to develop in association with specific killing (29,30). In the studies presented here, we found that AIDS patients had cytotoxic effector cells active against AIDS-LCL, and that the killing mediated by the cells could be enhanced significantly with IFN α. There was no evidence for restriction to autologous targets, and the cold target inhibition studies suggested that recognition and lysis of the

NK sensitive target, K562, was not affected by the presence of AIDS-LCL targets. We previously observed development and expression of cytotoxic activity in AIDS patients during the autologous mixed lymphocyte culture reaction, AMLR (20). This observation may have been analogous to the report of Palacios (31) that EBV increased the generation of CTL and NK in the AMLR. If so, this would be expected to occur in vivo during the development of AIDS.

The physiological significance of the findings reported here is unknown. It is well known that during the early stages of EBV infection, activation of T cells occurs. Such T cells would be susceptible to infection by retrovirus. If retrovirus is introduced, down regulation of T cell immunity would follow, leading to the establishment of unrestricted growth of EBV-infected B cells in vivo. The data presented here show that the proliferation of EBV positive B lymphocytes is not hindered by normal immunoregulatory mechanisms in AIDS, and that these cells produce very significant amounts of IFN α sufficient to have both physiological and immune regulatory effects. The sustained production of IFN α by B cells in AIDS could reflect concomittant infection with AIDS associated retrovirus. If so, the observation that patients with endogenous levels of serum IFN respond less well to exogenous IFN could reflect the difficulty of eliminating virus harbored by B cells. Data presented here suggest that AIDS patients' cytotoxicity toward infected B cells can be augmented in vitro and therefore might provide a basis for therapeutic intervention.

REFERENCES

1. M.S. Gottlieb, R. Schroff, H.M. Schanker, J.D. Weisman, P.T. Fan, R.A. Wolf, and A. Saxon, Pneumocystis carinii pneumonia and mucosal candidiasis in previously healthy homosexual men: Evidence of a new acquired cellular immunodeficiency, N. Engl. J. Med. 305:1425-1431 (1981).
2. H. Masur, M.A. Michelis, J.B. Greene, I. Onorato, R.A. Vande Sfouve, R.S. Holzman, G. Wormser, L. Brettman, M. Lange, and S. Cunningham-Rundles, A community acquired outbreak of Pneumocystis carinii pneumonia: initial manifestation of cellular immune dysfunction, N. Engl. J. Med. 305:1431-1438 (1981).
3. F.P. Siegal, C. Lopez, G.S. Hammer, A.E. Brown, S.J. Kornfeld, J. Gold, J. Hassett, S.Z. Hirschman, C. Cunningham-Rundles, B.R. Adelsbert, D.M. Parham, M. Siegal, S. Cunningham-Rundles, and D. Armstrong, Severe acquired immunodeficiency in male homosexuals manifested by chronic perianal ulcerative herpes simplex lesions, N. Engl. J. Med. 305:1439-1444 (1981).
4. H. Masur, M.A. Michelis, G.P. Wormser, S. Lewin, J. Gold, M.A. Tapper, J. Giron, C.W. Lerner, D. Armstrong, U. Setia, J.A. Sender, R.S. Siebken, P.Nicholas, F.P. Siegal, and S. Cunningham-Rundles, Previously healthy women with opportunistic infection vs. the initial manifestation of a community acquired cellular immunodeficiency extension of an emerging syndrome, Ann. Int. Med. 97:533-539 (1983).
5. J. Vieira, E. Frank, R.J. Spira, and S.H.Landesman, Acquired immune deficiency in Haitians: opportunistic infections in previously healthy Haitians, N. Engl. J. Med. 308:125-129 (1983).
6. J.H. Elliott, W.L.Hoppes, M.S. Platt, J.G. Thomas, I.P. Patel, and A. Gansar, The acquired immunodeficiency syndrome and Mycobacterium-avium intracellular bacteremia in a patient with hemophilia, Ann. Int. Med. 98:290-293 (1983).
7. J.L. Curran, P.N. Lawrence, H. Jaffe, J.E. Kaplan, L.D. Zyle, M. Chamberland, R. Weinstein, K.J. Lui, L.B. Schonberger, T.J. Spira, W.J. Alexander, G. Swinger, A. Amman, S. Solomon, D. Auerbach, D. Mildvan, R. Stoneburner, J.M. Jason, H.W. Haverkos, and B.L. Evatt, Acquired immunodeficiency syndrome (AIDS) associated with transfusions, N. Engl. J. Med. 310:69-75 (1984).

8. H.W. Jaffe, D.P. Frances, M.F. McLane, C. Cabradilla, J.W. Carran, B.W. Kilbourne, D.M. Lawrence, H.W. Haverkos, T.J. Spira, R.Y. Dodd, J. Gold, D. Armstrong, A. Ley, J. Groopman, J. Mullins, T.L. Lee, and M. Essex, Transfusion-associated AIDS: serologic evidence of human T-cell leukemia virus infection of donors, Science 223:1309-1311 (1984).
9. R.E. Stahl, A. Friedman-Kien, R. Dubin, M. Marmor, and S. Zolla-Pazner, Immunologic abnormalities in homosexual men. Relationship to Kaposi's sarcoma, Am. J. Med. 73:171-178 (1982).
10. S. Cunningham-Rundles, Analysis of cellular immune deficiency in acquired immunodeficiency syndrome, in: "The Acquired Immune Deficiency Syndrome and Infections of Homosexual Men," P. Ma and D. Armstrong, eds., Yorke, New York (1983).
11. C.E. Metroka, S. Cunningham-Rundles, M.S. Pollack, J.A. Sonnabend, J.M. Davis, B. Gordon, R.D. Fernandes, and J. Mouradian, Generalized lymphadenopathy in homosexual men, Ann. Int. Med. 99:585-591 (1982).
12. J.L. Ziegler, J.A. Beckslead, P.A. Volberding, D.I. Abrams, A.M. Levine, R.J. Lukes, P.S. Gill, R.L. Burkes, P.R. Meyer, C.E. Metroka, J. Mouradian, A. Moore, S.A. Riggs, J.J. Butler, F.C. Cabanillas, E. Hersh, G.R. Newell, L.J. Laubanstein, D. Knowles, C. Odajnyk, B. Raphael, B. Koziner, C. Urmacher, and B.D. Clarkson, Non-Hodgkins lymphoma in 90 homosexual men. Relation to generalized lymphadenopathy and the Acquired Immunodeficiency Syndrome, N. Engl. J. Med. 311:565-570 (1984).
13. A.M. Levine, P.B. Meyer, M.K. Begandy, J.W. Parker, C.R. Taylor, L. Irwin, and R.J. Lukes, Development of B cell lymphomas in homosexual men, Ann. Int. Med. 100:7-13 (1984).
14. Persistant, generalized lymphadenopathy among homosexual males, MMWR 31:249-251 (1982).
15. A. Ono, D.B. Amos, and H.S. Koren, Selective cellular natural killing against human leukaemic T cells and thymus, Nature 266:546-547 (1977).
16. S. Cunningham-Rundles, J.A. Hansen, and B. Dupont, Lymphocyte transformation to mitogens and antigens, in: "Clinical Immunobiology," Vol. 3, F. Bach and R.A. Good, eds., Academic Press, New York (1976).
17. S. Cunningham-Rundles, D. Filippa, P. Antonelli, D. Braun, and H. Ashikari, Natural killer cell activity of peripheral blood and regional lymph node lymphocytes in breast cancer, J. Nat. Can. Inst. 67:585-590 (1981).
18. S. Cunningham-Rundles, R.S. Bockman, and B.Y. Rubin, Modulation of natural cell-mediated cytotoxicity of T colonies and PBL by Interleukin-2, in: "Natural Cell-Mediated Immunity," pp. 415-420, R.B. Herberman, ed., Academic Press, New York (1982).
19. S.D. Hayward, L. Nogee, and G.S. Hayward, Organization of repeated regions within the Epstein-Barr virus DNA molecule, J. Virol. 33:507-521 (1980).
20. S. Cunningham-Rundles, B. Safai, C. Metroka, S.E. Krown, B.Y. Rubin, and W.E. Stahl, Lymphocyte effector function in vitro in the Acquired Immune Deficiency Syndrome, in: "AIDS: The Epidemic of Kaposi's Sarcoma and Opportunistic Infections," pp. 153-159, A.E. Friedman-Kien and L.J. Lauberstein, eds., Masson, USA (1984).
21. J.Y. Djeu, N. Stocks, K. Zoon, G.J. Stanton, T. Timonen, and R.B. Herberman, Positive selfrecognition of cytotoxicity in human natural killer cells by production of interferon upon exposure to influenza and herpes viruses, J. Exp. Med. 156:1222-1234 (1982).
22. C. Lopez, P.A. Fitzgerald, and F.P. Siegal, Severe Acquired Immune Deficiency Syndrome in male homosexuals: Diminished capacity to make interferon α in vitro associated with severe opportunistic infections, J. Infect. Dis. 148:962-966 (1983).
23. H.W. Murray, B.Y. Rubin, H. Masur, and R.B. Roberts, Impaired production of lymphokines and immune (gamma) interferon in the Acquired Immunodeficiency Syndrome, N. Engl. J. Med. 31:883-889 (1984).
24. S. Levin, T. Hahn, Z.T. Handzel, V. Bregman, N. Barzila, R. Myer, M. Tinowitz, E. Galili-Waisstub, and Z. Bentwich, Activated interferon system in healthy homosexuals, J. Clin. Immunol. (in press), (1984).

25. R.J. Melder and M. Ho, Modulation of natural killer cell activity in mice after interferon induction: depression of activity and depression of in vitro enhancement by interferon, Infect. Immun. 36:990-995 (1982).
26. S.H. Golub, F. Dorey, D. Hara, D.L. Morton, and M.W. Burk, Systemic administration of human leukocyte interferon to melanoma patients, J. Nat. Can. Inst. 68:703-710 (1982).
27. M. DeWaele, C. Thielemans, and B.K.G. Van Camp, Characterization of immunoregulatory T cells in EBV-induced infectious mononucleosis by monoclonal antibodies, N. Engl. J. Med. 304:460-462 (1981).
28. A.B. Rickinson, D.J. Moss, L. E. Wallace, M. Rowe, I.S. Misko, M.A. Epstein, and J.H. Pope, Long term T cell mediated immunity to Epstein-Barr virus, Can. Res. 41:4216-4221 (1981).
29. J. Seeley, E. Svedmyr, O. Weiland, G. Klein, E. Moller, E. Eriksson, K. Andersson, and L. Van der Waal, Epstein-Barr virus selective T cells in infectious mononucleosis are not restricted to HLA and B antigens, J. Immunol. 127:293-300 (1981).
30. Y. Tanaka, K. Sugamura, Y. Hinuma, H. Sato, and K. Okochi, Memory of Epstein-Barr virus specific cytotoxic T cells in normal seropositive adults as revealed by an in vitro restimulation method, J. Immunol. 125:1426-1431 (1980).
31. R. Palacios, Epstein-Barr virus increases the proliferative response and the generation of suppressor and cytotoxic T-cell functions in autologous mixed lymphocyte reaction, Scand. J. Immunol. 15:17-24 (1982).

ACKNOWLEDGMENTS

The authors gratefully acknowledge the technical assistance of Alison Hoppin, Desiree Ehleiter, Howard Block, and Helen Campbell and the help of Gail Dudley in preparation of the manuscript.

These studies were supported in part by N.Y. AO-163 and N.I.H. N.C.I. CA-34995.

EXPRESSION OF BETA 2 MICROGLOBULIN ON THE SURFACE OF MONONUCLEAR CELLS IN PATIENTS WITH ACQUIRED IMMUNE DEFICIENCY SYNDROME (AIDS) AND AIDS-RELATED COMPLEX (ARC)

Sudhir Gupta

Division of Basic and Clinical Immunology
University of California
Irvine, California 92717, U.S.A.

INTRODUCTION

Beta 2 microglobulin (B2-m) is a low molecular weight protein of 11,800 daltons and contains 100 amino acids. It was originally isolated from human urine and has been found in all body fluids (1-3). B2-m shows a homology with CH3 domain of immunoglobulin molecules and is associated with class I major histocompatibility complex molecules. B2-m is present on the surface of and synthesized by virtually all somatic cells. In vitro, both normal and malignant human cell lines and activated normal lymphocytes synthesize B2-m (4, 5). B2-m has been shown to play a role in T cell response to mitogens, soluble antigens and alloantigens (6-12). Acquired immune deficiency syndrome (AIDS) is characterized by several defects of T cell functions and clinically manifested by opportunistic infections and/or Kaposi's sarcoma (KS) (13-16). Recently, increased plasma levels of B2-m in patients with AIDS and hemophilia have been described (17-19). In this study we have examined the expression of surface B2-m on the mononuclear cells (MNC) from patients with AIDS and AIDS-related complex (ARC), using a monoclonal antibody and fluorescence-activated cell sorter analyzer (20).

MATERIALS AND METHODS

Ten patients with AIDS, 15 with AIDS-related complex (ARC), 10 asymptomatic homosexuals, and 13 healthy heterosexuals were the subjects of the study. Diagnosis of AIDS was confirmed according to surveillance definition criteria of the Center for Disease Control (21). Patients with ARC presented with prolonged generalized persistent lymphadenopathy, low-grade fever, night sweats and showed cutaneous anergy to recall antigens, and depressed proliferative response to mitogens.

Mononuclear cells (MNC) were separated on Ficoll-Hypaque density gradient. Cells were washed three times and resuspended in phosphate buffer saline. Cells were mixed with appropriate dilution of monoclonal antibody against B2-m for 30 minutes at 4°C. Cells were washed and counted with FACS analyzer. In order to measure the proportions of high intensity B2-m+ cells, gates were set between 90-200 channels. Data are presented as both percent and absolute numbers of B2-m+ cells. Analysis was performed by student "t" test.

RESULTS

The results of the proportion and number of high density B2-m+ MNC are shown in Table 1. The proportions of high density B2-m+ cells (mean ± SD) in patients with AIDS (54.8 ± 7.4) and ARC (54.0 ± 8.0) were significantly lower ($p < 0.05$) than those of asymptomatic homosexuals (73.0 ± 6.5) and healthy heterosexuals (75.0 ± 7.0). The absolute numbers of high density B2-m+ MNC were significantly decreased in AIDS (222 ± 34, $p < 0.001$) and ARC (998 ± 274, $p < 0.05$) when compared to asymptomatic homosexuals (1595 ± 328) and healthy heterosexuals (1625 ± 677).

Table 1. Proportions and Numbers of High Density B2-m+ MNC in AIDS and ARC

High Density B2-m+ MNC	AIDS	ARC	Asymptomatic Homosexuals	Healthy Heterosexuals
PROPORTIONS (Mean ± SD)	54.8 ± 7.4	54.0 ± 8.0	73.0 ± 6.5	75.0 ± 7.0
P value	< 0.05	< 0.05	---	---
ABSOLUTE NUMBERS (per mm^3)	222 ± 34	998 ± 274	1595 ± 328	1625 ± 677
P value	< 0.001	< 0.05	---	---

Data of the proportions and numbers of total (both high and low density) B2-m+ MNC in AIDS and ARC are given in Table 2. The proportions of B2-m+ MNC were comparable in all the four groups; however, the absolute numbers of total B2-m+ MNC were significantly ($p < 0.001$) decreased in AIDS when compared with asymptomatic homosexuals and healthy heterosexuals. The absolute number of B2-m+ MNC in ARC was also decreased, but the differences from asymptomatic homosexuals or healthy heterosexuals were not significant ($p > 0.05$).

Table 2. Proportions and Numbers of Total (High and Low Density) B2-m+ MNC in AIDS and ARC

Total B2-m+ MNC	AIDS	ARC	Asymptomatic Homosexuals	Healthy Heterosexuals
PROPORTIONS (mean ± SD)	92.8 ± 3.2	94.4 ± 2.8	98.3 ± 4.2	97.6 ± 2.8
P value	NS[a]	NS	---	---
ABSOLUTE NUMBERS (per mm^3)	394 ± 52	1792 ± 144	2201 ± 232	1942 ± 235
P value	< 0.001	NS	---	---

[a]NS = Not significant

DISCUSSION

This study demonstrates significantly reduced levels of high density B2-m+ MNC in patients with AIDS and ARC when compared with asymptomatic male homosexuals and healthy heterosexuals. The changes in high density B2-m+ MNC appear to be due to a shift from high density to low density B2-m+ MNC (20). A significant correlation has been observed between the deficiency of B2-m+ MNC and the abnormal ratios of Leu 3+/Leu 2+ T cells in AIDS (20). In the AIDS group, no difference was observed with regard to deficiency of B2-m+ MNC, among those with opportunistic infections and those with Kaposi's sarcoma (data not shown).

B2-m is a low molecular weight protein present on virtually all somatic cells and appears to play a role in certain T cell functions (1-3, 6-12). Therefore a deficiency of high density B2-m+ cells could be responsible (at least in part) for certain T cell defects in AIDS and ARC. The density of B2-m on the surface of a cell appears to be determined by the rate of its secretion from cell surface into serum. Malignant human lymphoma cell lines have been shown to express lower amounts of B2-m as compared to normal lymphocytes. Azocar et al (22) have reported that *in vitro* activated lymphocytes express less amounts of B2-m than the resting cells. In AIDS, B lymphocytes have been shown to be activated *in vivo* (23). This could result in increased turnover of the surface membrane B2-m resulting in decreased expression of high density B2-m in AIDS and ARC. Alternatively, attrition of surface of T cells (possibly due to infection by HTLV III) could result in shedding of bits of B2-m in the serum. This might also explain elevated plasma levels of B2-m observed in AIDS (17, 19). Purified gamma interferon has been shown to increase the synthesis and expression of both class I and II MHC antigens (24, 25). In AIDS, gamma interferon production is deficient (26), which could be responsible for decreased B2-m synthesis and therefore deficiency of high density B2-m+ MNC in AIDS.

Studies are in progress to investigate *in vitro* synthesis of B2-m by T cell subsets, B cells and macrophages in patients with AIDS and ARC to understand the precise mechanism(s) for deficiency of high density B2-m+ MNC. Longitudinal studies will be required to determine if this deficiency of B2-m+ MNC could be used as an early marker for AIDS or for predicting the progression to ARC or AIDS in high risk group individuals.

ACKNOWLEDGMENTS

This work was supported by a grant from USPHS-AI-20717 and the University of California Systemwide Task Force on AIDS.

REFERENCES

1. B. Berggard, L. Bjorck, R. Gigen, and L. Logdberg, β_2-microglobulin, *Scand J Clin Lab Invest* 40 (Supp. 154):13 (1980).
2. F.A. Karlsson, L. Wibell, and P.E. Erin, β_2-microglobulin in clinical medicine, *Scand J Clin Lab Invest* 40 (Supp. 140):27 (1980).
3. M.D. Paulik and R.A. Reisfeld, β_2-microglobulin, *Contemp Topics Mol Immunol* 4:157 (1975).

4. K. Nilsson, P.E. Evrin, I. Berggard, and J. Ponten, Involvement of lymphoid and non-lymphoid cells in the production of β_2 microglobulin--a homologue of the constant domain of IgG, Nature (New Biol) 244:44 (1973).
5. G.M. Bernier and M.W. Fanger, Synthesis of β_2-microglobulin by stimulated lymphocytes, J Immunol 109:407, 1972.
6. M.L. Bach, S.W. Huang, R. Hong, and M.D. Paulik, β_2-microglobulin association with lymphocyte receptors, Science 182:1350 (1973).
7. J.B. Lindblom, L. Ostberg, and P.A. Peterson, β_2-microglobulin on the cell surface. Relationship to HLA-antigens and the mixed leukocyte culture reaction, Tissue Antigens 4:186 (1974).
8. R.T. McCalmon, R.T. Kurbo, and H.M. Grey, Inhibition of anti-β_2-microglobulin antisera of responder cells and not of stimulator cells in the mixed lymphocyte reaction, Scand J Immunol 4:613 (1975).
9. B.G. Solheim, Association between β_2m-HLA molecule and membrane structures responsible for lymphocyte activation, Transplant Rev 21:35 (1974).
10. L. Logdberg, R. Cigen, and I. Berggard, Effects of anti-guinea pig β_2-microglobulin antibodies on lymphocyte transformation induced by specific antigens or mitogens, Scand J Immunol 9:263 (1979).
11. R.T. McCalmon, R.T. Kubo, and H.M. Grey, Effect of anti-β_2-microglobulin on antigen and allogeneic lymphocyte-induced proliferation of human lymphocytes. J Immunol 114:1766 (1975).
12. C. Vincent, M. Robert, and J.P. Revillard, Effects of anti-β_2-microglobulin antibodies on human lymphocytes, Cell Immunol 18:152 (1975).
13. A.J. Ammann, D. Abram, M. Conant, D. Chudwing, M. Cowan, P. Volberding, B. Lewis, and C. Casavant, Acquired immune deficiency in homosexual men: Immunologic profile, Clin Immunol Immunopath 27:315 (1983).
14. R.W. Schroft, M.S. Gottlieb, H.E. Prince, L.L. Chai, and J.H. Fahey, Immunological studies of homosexual men with immunodeficiency and Kaposi's sarcoma, Clin Immunol Immunopath 27:300 (1983).
15. S. Gupta and B. Safai, Deficient autologous mixed lymphocyte reaction in Kaposi's sarcoma associated with deficiency of Leu 3+ responder T cells, J Clin Invest 71:296 (1983).
16. S. Gupta, S. Gillis, M. Thornton, and M. Goldberg, Autologous mixed lymphocyte reaction in man. XIV. Deficiency of the autologous mixed lymphocyte reaction in acquired immune deficiency syndrome (AIDS) and AIDS-related complex (ARC): In vitro effect of purified interleukin-1 and interleukin-2, Clin Exp Immunol 58:395 (1984).
17. R.B. Bhalla, B. Safai, R. Mertelsman, and M.K. Schwartz, Abnormal high concentrations of beta 2 microglobulin in acquired immunodeficiency syndrome (AIDS) patients, (Letter) Clin Chem 29:1560 (1983).
18. J.K. Kreiss, D.N. Lawrence, C.K. Kasper, A.L. Goldstein, P.H. Naylor, M.F. McLane, T-H. Lee, and M. Essex, Antibody to human T-cell leukemia virus membrane antigens, beta$_2$-microglobulin levels, and thymosin alpha 1 levels in hemophiliacs and their spouses, Ann Int Med 100:178 (1984).
19. P. Francioli and F. Clement, Beta$_2$-microglobulin and immunodeficiency in a homosexual man (Letter) New Engl J Med 307:1402 (1982).

20. S. Gupta, Monoclonal antibody-defined β_2-microglobulin positive mononuclear cells in AIDS, Scand J Immunol, in press.
21. R.M. Selik, H.W. Haverkos, and J.W. Curran, Acquired immune deficiency syndrome (AIDS) trends in the United States 1978-1982, Amer J Med 76:493 (1984).
22. J. Azocar, M. Essex, A. Watson, E. Gazit, D. Anderson, and E.J. Yuris, Changes in the expression of HLA and β_2-microglobulin by cultured lymphoid cells, Human Immunol 5:283 (1982).
23. H.C. Lane, H. Masur, L.C. Edgar, G. Whalen, A.H. Rook, and A.S. Fauci, Abnormalities of B cell activation and immunoregulation in patients with the acquired immunodeficiency syndrome, New Engl J Med 309:453 (1983).
24. J.L. Virelizier, N. Perez, F. Arenzana-Seisdedos, and R. Devos, Pure interferon gamma enhances class II HLA antigens of human monocyte cell lines, Eur J Immunol 14:106 (1984).
25. D. Wallach, M. Fellous, and M. Revel, Preferential effect of interferon on the synthesis of HLA antigens and their mRNAs in human cells, Nature 299:833 (1982).
26. H.W. Murray, B.Y. Rubin, H. Hasur, and R.B. Roberts, Impaired production of lymphokines and immune (gamma) interferon in the acquired immunodeficiency syndrome, New Engl J Med 310:883 (1984).

ISOLATED THROMBOCYTOPENIA IN HOMOSEXUAL MEN - LONGITUDINAL FOLLOW-UP

Donald I. Abrams, Dobri D. Kiprov and
Paul A. Volberding
AIDS Clinic, San Francisco General Hospital
and Children's Hospital of San Francisco
San Francisco, California

One of the most clinically challenging, yet infrequently discussed, of the AIDS-associated syndromes is the problem of immune thrombocytopenic purpura (ITP). ITP is a diagnosis more frequently encountered in its acute form in children following viral infections and in its chronic presentation in middle-aged women. Morris et al published their account of auto-immune thrombocytopenic purpura in homosexual men in June 1984(1). Their manuscript described a cluster of ITP in 12 homosexual men with backgrounds similar to those recognized in patients with acquired immunodeficiency syndrome. Subsequently the problem has also been recognized in narcotics addicts and hemophiliacs without other manifestations of AIDS(2,3). To date, 32 homosexual men with isolated thrombocytopenia of immune origin have been evaluated in the AIDS Clinic at San Francisco General Hospital. Our experience with this group constitutes the basis of the following discussion.

Thrombocytopenia itself is a recognized complication of many of the confirmed AIDS diagnoses. A percentage of our patients with Kaposi's sarcoma are noted either at the time of diagnosis or during treatment to develop low platelet counts(4). A similar phenomenon has been seen in those patients diagnosed with AIDS-related lymphomas. Patients with Pneumocystis pneumonia may present with mild thrombocytopenia at the time of their initial diagnosis. However, it is more common for thrombocytopenia to develop during the course of treatment for this opportunistic infection (5). Often the platelet count lowers to an alarming level with dramatic rapidity. This is generally assumed to be drug-induced thrombocytopenia. The majority of our patients who have been tested at the time of their thrombocytopenia during antibiotic treatment have demonstrated platelet-associated immunoglobulin. Mild platelet count depression to the 100,000 to 150,000 ul range has been found in approximately 5% of patients undergoing evaluation for the syndrome of persistent generalized lymphadenopathy in our clinic(6). Thrombocytopenia associated with other features of the lymphadenopathy syndrome appears to be associated with an increased risk of progression from lymphadenopathy syndrome to bona fide AIDS in our natural history study(7). Although one-quarter of the patients evaluated for the problem of isolated thrombocytopenia without other manifestations of AIDS did have peripheral lymphadenopathy on physical examination, the magnitude of their thrombocytopenia justified their inclusion in the ITP cohort.

The demographic backgrounds of the 32 homosexual men with isolated thrombocytopenia evaluated in our clinic are similar to those of AIDS patients(8). The mean and median age of the group is 33 years. Twenty-nine men are Caucasian with 3 ITP patients of Hispanic origin. One patient was diagnosed with ITP in 1980, 5 in 1982, and 17 in 1983. There was an apparent cluster of 14 of the 1983 cases diagnosed in the four-month period from April until August. The significance of this seasonal variation is unclear. The same pattern was demonstrated in cases diagnosed in 1984.

The clinical presentation of patients with isolated thrombocytopenia has been generally benign. No patient has suffered major gastrointestinal or central nervous system bleeds during the course of follow-up. Six patients denied any antecedent bleeding prior to their diagnosis of ITP which was made on routine hematologic problems performed for unrelated reasons. Easy bruising with ecchymoses and petechiae were reported in over half of the patients. Five patients noted gum bleeding, 3 rectal bleeding, 2 epistaxis, and 2 patients sought medical attention for blood in their seminal ejaculate leading to the diagnosis of ITP. The mean duration from onset of symptoms to the diagnosis of ITP in this group has been one month.

Initial laboratory findings in the cohort of patients with isolated thrombocytopenia revealed a platelet count of 20,000/ul (range 3000 to 55,000). A mild degree of anemia (Hct. 37 to 40%) was found in only 3 of 32 patients evaluated. White blood cell counts averaged 6600/ul. The absence of anemia or leukopenia defined these patients has having isolated thrombocytopenia. Numerous patients with AIDS or prodomal symptoms have presented to our clinic with pancytopenia. Although these patients may also demonstrate platelet-associated immunoglobulin on testing, patients demonstrating pancytopenia are not included in this ITP cohort discussion.

Bone marrow examinations in patients with isolated thrombocytopenia have revealed adequate to increased megakaryocytes in 25 patients studied. Platelet-associated immunoglobulin was detected in all members of this cohort. Anti-lymphocyte antibodies were also present in the majority of patients(9).

Lymphocyte subset abnormalities are common in patients with auto-immune phenomenon such as immune thrombocytopenic purpura. Normally, in such situations, the helper cell population is increased yielding a T-lymphocyte helper-to-suppressor ratio greater than normal. The patients in this study demonstrated a mean of 1700 lymphocytes/ul (range 800 to 3100). A marked decrease in both number and percentage of

OKT4 positive lymphocytes was found in patients with AIDS-related ITP. The mean OKT4 number was 390 per cu/mm with an OKT4 percentage of 18%. Suppressor cells were increased to a mean of 1200/ul with a percentage of 51%. The resultant mean OKT4:OKT8 ratio in this group was depressed to 0.4 (mean 0.1 to 0.8). This again is an unexpected phenotype in patients with auto-immune phenomena and supports the contention that ITP in homosexual men is likely related to infection with the putative AIDS retrovirus. Serologic studies of antibody to HTLV-III in this cohort performed by Dr. Robert Gallo in conjunction with Dr. James Goedert confirmed this contention(10).

Karpatkin working with the New York Group that originally described the problem of auto-immune thrombocytopenia in homosexual men, has suggested that the mechanism of thrombocytopenia in AIDS-related ITP is secondary to circulating immune complexes precipitating on the platelets(11). In our cohort, circulating immune complexes were detected in approximately one-half of the patients evaluated via the Clq assay. Stricker of the Cancer Research Institute at the University of California at San Francisco has demonstrated via a western blot technique a unique antibody in the sera of patients with AIDS-related ITP(12). This protein appears to be targeted against a specific platelet antigen of molecular weight 25,000. This unique antibody has not been found in high frequency in patients with non-AIDS-related immune thrombocytopenia. Continued investigation as to whether AIDS-related immune thrombocytopenia is secondary to an innocent bystander phenomenon or direct anti-platelet antibodies is ongoing at this time.

Perhaps the most challenging aspect of the clinical management of patients with AIDS-related ITP has been investigating therapeutic modalities. Even in our earliest cases, the possibility that thrombocytopenia might somehow be associated with the immunosuppression seen in AIDS, made the use of steroids of some concern(13,14). However, to date, 20 patients with AIDS-related ITP have undergone prednisone therapy(8,15). Most of these patients were diagnosed prior to 1984. Prednisone was prescribed at a dosage of 1 mg/kg per day for an initial three week period with subsequent tapering. The results of steroid therapy in our cohort of AIDS-related ITP patients yielded only two patients obtaining sustained remissions of their thrombocytopenia. A third patient underwent 6 months of steroid therapy. At the time his treatment was discontinued his platelet count had risen to 90,000/ul. Over the ensuing year, without any further therapeutic intervention, his platelet count returned to normal. The majority of patients begun on prednisone demonstrated a rise in their platelet count during the initial three week high-dose bolus. Eight additional patients achieved normal platelet counts during the initial therapy which subsequently fell to pretreatment levels as the dosage was tapered. An additional 8 patients obtained significant increases in their platelet count, yet failed to reach normal values during steroid therapy. Only 2 patients demonstrated no response to their initial three week course of prednisone.

None of the patients treated with steroids suffered an

episode of opportunistic infection or malignant transformation while on therapy. The complications of treatment were similar to those described in patients without AIDS on prolonged steroid courses. Weight gain and moon facies developed in 15 of 20 patients treated. Fourteen patients developed oral Candida while on treatment. One of these patients, however, was noted to have thrush prior to the institution of steroids which was exacerbated with therapy. Marked dysphoric reactions described as an intense sense of "speeding" were described by 10 patients during the course of their steroids. Steroid acne and activation of herpes labialis were also seen in 10 of the 20 patients. One patient developed a severe proximal muscle weakness of the lower extremities that was felt by neurology consultants to be the result of a steroid myopathy. Another patient with a past history of treatment for pulmonary tuberculosis 20 years prior to developing his ITP, experienced an episode of headache and fever after six months of prednisone therapy. Cerebrospinal fluid examination revealed a monocytosis with negative cultures. Repeat lumbar puncture three weeks later when the symptomatology had abated was negative. It was presumed that this episode represented a self-limited aseptic meningitis.

Serial helper-to-suppressor lymphocyte ratios have been performed on patients initiating prednisone therapy(15). A mild decrease in total lymphocyte count was appreciated in patients treated with prednisone. An equivalent decrease was noted in both the OKT4 and OKT8 population during steroid therapy. This yielded no signficant change from the baseline helper-to-suppressor ratio in these patients. These trends were reversed on tapering off prednisone therapy. In the ITP patients treated with steroids who had associated peripheral lymphadenopathy on physical examination, the nodes became impalpable during treatment. As these patients were tapered off of steroids, the generalized lymphadenopathy was again appreciable.

Splenectomy has been performed on 12 patients with AIDS-related ITP. In 2 patients this was the initial modality of therapy. The remaining 10 underwent splenectomy after failing steroid trials. Eight of the 12 patients splenectomized achieved sustained remissions with normal platelet counts postoperatively. Three of the surgical failures were noted to be thrombocytopenic within one month of their splenectomy. The fourth patient was followed with a normal platelet count for four months postoperatively until dropping his platelet count to 30,000. Again, serial helper-to-suppressor lymphocyte evaluations revealed no change in the ratio following splenectomy. However, a fivefold increase in total lymphocytes occurred, distributed among both OKT4 and OKT8 subsets.

Additional therapeutic modalities which have been employed in patients with AIDS-related ITP seen in our clinic have been the use of danazol and vincristine. Neither of these agents appear to have efficacy in producing sustained normalization of thrombocytopenia. Nor did danazol, in conjunction with prednisone therapy, appear to have any effect on normalization of the reversed helper-to-suppressor ratio.

Immune thrombocytopenia is now recognized as an AIDS-related condition. Similar to the situation with the lymphadenopathy syndrome, it has been presumed that patients demonstrating thrombocytopenia are expressing an alternative phenotypic response to infection with the AIDS retrovirus. Patients have been comforted by the notion that thrombocytopenia would most likely be their only manifestation of infection. However, 2 patients in this cohort have developed additional complications. One of these patients received one year of steroid therapy before he underwent successful splenectomy. Three years following the onset of his ITP, the patient was evaluated for fevers, abdominal complaints, and an elevated erythrocyte sedimentation rate. He was discovered to have a small bowel lymphoma. His platelet count was normal at the time of his malignant diagnosis. A second patient treated with three months of steroids followed by splenectomy has now been treated for Pneumocystis carinii pneumonia thirty-one months after his initial ITP diagnosis. A third patient has been evaluated for possible Pneumocystis with a negative bronchoscopy. He continues to have pulmonary symptoms, intermittent fevers, an elevated erythrocyte sedimentation rate and positive Gallium scan for diffuse pulmonary parenchymal uptake. His initial diagnosis of ITP was made thirteen months ago. The mean duration of follow-up for the cohort is 18 months. In view of the fact that 2 patients have progressed to more severe manifestations 31 and 36 months following their ITP diagnoses, the possibility exists that presentation with isolated thrombocytopenia may, in fact, be a harbinger of a more serious AIDS diagnosis in the future.

At the present time, patients referred for evaluation of isolated thrombocytopenia are apprised of the success rates of the various therapeutic interventions in the existent cohort. With the 10% complete response rate and the high incidence of disturbing, though not life-threatening side effects, most patients have not elected a steroid trial. Splenectomy is recommended as initial treatment for patients willing to accept the surgical procedure. Most new patients have elected careful observation without therapeutic intervention. To date, no serious adverse bleeding episodes have been recorded in the untreated group despite platelet counts as low as 10,000. A protocol to explore the role of plasma exchange and plasmapheresis employing a Staph protein A column for immuno-adsorption is currently being evaluated.

Supported in part by a grant from the Universitywide Task Force on AIDS, University of California

REFERENCES

1. Morris L. Distenfeld A, Amorosi E, and Karpatkin S. Autoimmune thrombocytopenic purpura in homosexual men. Ann Int Med 96(Part I):714-717, 1984.
2. Savona S, Nardi M, and Karpatkin S. Thrombocytopenic purpura in narcotics addicts. Blood 64:240a, 1984 (abstract).
3. Brettler DB, Szymanski IO, Sullivan JL, et al. Platelet associated IgG in hemophilia. Blood 64:240a, 1984 (abstract).

4. Abrams DI, Chinn EK, Lewis BJ, et al. Hematologic manifestations in homosexual men with Kaposi's sarcoma. Am J Clin Pathol 81:13-18, 1984.
5. Jaffe HS, Ammann AJ, Abrams DI, Lewis BJ, and Golden JA. Complications of co-trimoxazole in treatment of AIDS-associated Pneumocystis carinii pneumonia in homosexual men. Lancet ii:1109-1111, 1983.
6. Abrams DI, Lewis BJ, Beckstead JH, Casavant CA and Drew WL. Persistent diffuse lymphadenopathy in homosexual men: Endpoint or prodrome? Ann Int Med 100:801-808, 1984.
7. Abrams DI. Lymphadenopathy in homosexual men. IN: Advances in Host Defences, Vol. 4, Gallin J and Fauci A, eds., Raven Press, 1985. In press.
8. Abrams DI, Volberding PA, Linker CA, et al. Immune thrombocytopenic purpura in homosexual men: Clinical manifestations and treatment results. Blood 62:108a, 1983 (abstract).
9. Kiprov DD, Morand P, Moss A, Sherman JC and Spira T. Correlation of antilymphocyte bodies (ALA) with seropositivity for lymphadenopathy virus (LAV). Proceedings of International Conference on Acquired Immunodeficiency Syndrome, 1985 (submitted).
10. Abrams DI, Kiprov DD, Goedert MG, et al. HTLV-III antibodies and development of AIDS in homosexual men presenting with immune thrombocytopenia. Proceedings of International Conference on Acquired Immunodeficiency Syndrome, 1985 (submitted).
11. Walsh CM, Nardi MA, and Karpatkin S. On the mechanism of thrombocytopenic purpura in sexually active homosexual men. N Engl J Med 311:635-639, 1984.
12. Stricker RB, Abrams DI, Corash L and Shuman MA. Target platelet antigen in AIDS-related immune thrombocytopenia. Blood 64:241a, 1984 (abstract).
13. Saxon A, Stevens RH, Ramer SJ, Clements PJ, and Yu DTY. Glucocorticoids administered in vivo inhibit human suppressor T lymphocyte function and diminish B lymphocyte responsiveness in in vitro immunoglobulin synthesis. J Clin Invest Vol. 61:922-930, 1977.
14. Zweiman B, Atkins PC, Bedard PM, Flaschen SL and Lisak RP. Corticosteroid effects on circulating lymphocyte subset levels in normal humans. J Clin Immunol 4:151-155, 1984.
15. Abrams D, Kiprov D, Stricker R, and Volberding P. Prednisone therapy in AIDS-related immune thrombocytopenia (ITP): Clinical, hematologic and immunologic consequences. Proceedings American Society of Clinical Oncology (ASCO) 1985 (submitted).

ORAL VIRAL LEUKOPLAKIA - A NEW AIDS-ASSOCIATED CONDITION

John S. Greenspan,
Deborah Greenspan,
Evelyne T. Lennette,
Donald I. Abrams,
Marcus A. Conant, and
Vibeke H. Petersen

Schools of Dentistry and Medicine and AIDS Clinical Research Center, University of California San Francisco and Virolab Emeryville, CA

INTRODUCTION

Viral leukoplakia of the tongue in immunosuppressed male homosexuals (oral "hairy" leukoplakia, H.L.) is a newly described lesion showing an association with the subsequent development of AIDS, often with Pneumocystis carinii pneumonia. The lesion appears to contain papillomavirus as well as a second virus of the herpes-group (1). In this paper we present evidence for the presence, within the epithelial cells of hairy leukoplakia, of both papillomavirus and Epstein-Barr virus (EBV), and for the presence of EB viral capsid antigen (VCA).

PATIENTS AND METHOD

Patients

The patient population has been described previously (1) and consists of referrals to the oral medicine clinic at the University of California, San Francisco from the UCSF AIDS Clinical Research Center or by physicians and dentists in the San Francisco area. Patients gave medical and social histories in response to standard questionnaires and had complete physical and oral examinations. When oral white lesions were found, they were subjected to smear and culture for Candida as well as to biopsy when patients' permission was granted.

Oral biopsy

Incisional biopsy specimens were obtained from selected cases of HL under local anaesthesia. Routine histopathology and periodic acid/Schiff (PAS) staining was performed on formal-saline-fixed, paraffin-embedded samples. Frozen samples for viral immunostaining and DNA hybridization were obtained from the biopsy specimens. Samples for electron microscopy were fixed with 3% glutaldehyde, postfixed in 1% buffered osmic acid and embedded in epon. Thin sections were stained with lead citrate. A total of 60 HL biopsies were obtained. Due to the limited size of the specimens, only papillomavirus antigen staining was attempted on all of the specimens. Where available, remaining portions of the tissues were sufficient for assignment at most to only one additional testing procedure. Of 60 HL specimens, 20 were stained for EBV antigen and electron microscopy examination was done on 23 specimens. For 6 of the 20 HL patients whose lesional specimens were stained for EBV, biopsies of normal buccal mucosa were also obtained for testing. Additional appropriate control specimens were collected for each procedure as follows. For the staining of papilloma-virus antigen, control biopsies were paraffin embedded biopsies from 10 oral warts or condylomata (positive controls), 5 cases of epithelial hyperplasia, 3 of lichen planus and 2 of fibroepithelial hyperplasia. For the staining of herpesviruses, control frozen biopsies were from oral mucosa lesions of 2 cases of pemphigoid, 1 of pemphigus, 2 of erythema multiforme, 2 of epithelial hyperplasia, 2 of epithelial dysplasia and 2 of lichen planus.

Papillomavirus antigen

Peroxidase-anti-peroxidase (PAP) immunocytochemistry for papillomavirus core antigen (HPV) was performed as described previously (1). In addition to the control biopsies described above, controls for the staining reagents included human fetal diploid lung cells infected with herpes simplex 1 & 2 (HSV 1 & HSV 2), with cytomegalovirus (CMV), with varicella-zoster virus (VZV) and a lymphoma (P3HR1) EBV-producer cell line.

EBV Serology

Antibodies to EB viral capsid antigen (VCA), to the early antigen-diffuse component (EA-D) and early antigen-restricted component (EA-R) were measured by the method of Henle et al. (2). Antibodies to EB-associated nuclear antigen (EBNA) were measured by the anti-complement indirect immunofluorescence assay (ACIF) using guinea pig complement and fluorescein-isothiocyanate conjugated (FITC) rabbit anti-guinea pic C3 (3). In addition to sera collected from 30 HL patients, controls included sera from 10 apparently healthy male homosexuals and 10 heterosexual males (5 healthy and 5 with recurrent apthous ulcers).

Tissue staining for the Herpesviruses

Cryostat sections (5 um thick) from HL and control patients were stained by a direct immunofluorescence assay to detect HSV 1 & 2, and VZV using FITC-rabbit hyperimmune sera. For CMV and EBV antigens, the ACIF procedure was applied as described previously (4), using human sera with the following specificities: 3 sera were EBV+/CMV-, 3 sera were CMV+/EBV- and 1 EBV-/CMV-. In addition, EBNA negative sera from 3 infectious mononucleosis (IM) patients who were CMV negative were used to determine the EBV antigens found in the HL biopsies. Serum A is VCA+/EA-, serum B is VCA+/D+/R-, serum C is VCA+/D-/R+.

Immunological studies

Delayed hypersensitivity skin testing and the assessment of T_4 and T_8 numbers, as well as the T_4/T_8 ratio of peripheral blood lymphocytes were performed as described previously (1).

RESULTS

Clinical

Between October 1981 and November 1984, 77 cases of HL were diagnosed, including the 37 previously reported (1). The clinical appearances of the lesions were as we have described and no further cases involving mucosa other than the tongue have been seen. 70 cases did not have AIDS, according to the Centers for Disease Control definition (5) at the time of biopsy. 7 cases did show features of AIDS at the time of diagnosis of HL, of these 1 had *Pneumocystic carinii* pneumonia, 6 had Kaposi's sarcoma. Of 70 cases without AIDS at the time of diagnosis of HL, 15 have developed AIDS. These included 12 cases of PCP of whom 2 have died, 1 case of KS and 2 of other life threatening opportunistic infections, of whom one has died. Of the remaining 56 cases, 54 are without AIDS while 2 have been lost to follow-up. The 15 cases of AIDS developed at 1,1,1,1,2,2,3,3,5,5,8,10,17,27 and 31 months from the time of HL diagnosis.

Histopathology

Biopsy specimens for diagnosis were obtained from 64 patients. All showed the histological appearances of HL described previously (1). These resemble those of the flat wart of skin and are remarkable for three features in particular; fine keratin projections in many cases; koilocytosis of prickle cells and little if any subepithelial inflammatory cell infiltration. Mild atypia was seen in 7 cases.

Immunological findings

Of 57 patients, showing no features of AIDS at the time of diagnosis of HL, and skin tested with the four antigens PPD, candida, mumps and trichophytin, 20 showed no response, 14 responded to only one antigen, 21 to two antigens, 2 to three and none to all four. Of 25 of the same group of non-AIDS HL patients whose T_4/T_8 ratio was assessed, 23 showed a ratio of less than 1 while all 25 had a ratio of less than 1.3.

Candida was found in smear and culture from a scraping of the lesion in 47 of 77 cases and was also found in PAS-stained sections in 30 of 64 from whom biopsy specimens were taken. We have again found regression of the lesion after antifungal therapy in very few cases (6/47).

Ultrastructure

Examination of specimens from 23 cases, involving the viewing of at least 150 epithelial cells, revealed in each case examples of prickle cells showing individual structures with appearances somewhat resembling previous descriptions of individual papillomavirus particles (6-7). These took the form of polygonal particles approximately 46-52 nm in diameter and containing a poorly defined internal structure. These were found only within nuclei and in small numbers (2 to 18 per nucleus). Typical arrays of papillomavirus particles (8) were not seen. 17 of the same 23 samples showed numerous particles of the herpes-type virus described previously (1). These were 100 nm naked capsids within prickle cell nuclei, accompanied by numerous arrays of ill-defined particles 65-75 nm in diameter in 9 cases. Enveloped virions 150-200 nm in diameter were present in the cytoplasm and in the intercellular spaces.

Papillomavirus antigen

Of 60 HL biopsy specimens tested, 43 (71.7%) showed positive staining. Six of 10 oral warts and condylomata (60%), none of the 10 other oral mucosal lesions and none of the 6 non-lesional buccal mucosa specimens from HL cases showed positive staining. Cell lines containing the herpes group viruses were all negative.

Herpesviridae antigens

Direct immunofluorescence staining was negative on cryosections for HSV 1 & 2 and for VZV. ACIF staining for CMV using 3 reference CMV+/EBV- sera were uniformly negative. No staining were obtained with any of the 4 EBV- sera. Control non-HL biopsies were uniformly negative for any member of the herpesvirus group.

Staining for EBV was consistently positive and striking in appearance. Nineteen of 20 specimens showed intense nuclear staining in epithelial cells with each of the 6 EBV+ reference sera. EB positive staining cells in HL biopsies were confined to the prickle and koilocytotic cell layer. On cryostat sections, the positive cells appeared as a well defined ribbon of fluorescence, usually less than 6 to 8 cells deep. In 6 patients from whom both lesion (tongue) and non-lesion (buccal) tissues were available, positive EBV staining was seen in 5 of 6 patients and in the lesions only. Interestingly, EM examinations of the specimens from the EBV-negative HL cases showed only papillomavirus-like particles.

We further identified the EBV antigen seen in the sections to be predominantly VCA, as IM serum A, with antibodies to VCA only, produced the characteristic intense staining. IM serum B (VCA+/D+) produced an additional, but subtler staining pattern. Many of the brightly positive nuclei showed a halo of speckled staining, characteristic of D antigen staining seen in all EA positive lymphoblastoid cells.

EBV-Serology

The results of the EB serology revealed a sharp difference in geometric mean (GM) anti-VCA titers between heterosexuals (GM 367) and healthy homosexuals (GM 1778). There was aproximately a 5 fold difference in the mean titers between the two groups. The HL patients appear to be a subgroup of the homosexual donors, as their anti-VCA titers (GM 2189) were noticeably higher than either of the two control groups.

DISCUSSION

Epstein-Barr virus is associated with several clinical entities involving at least two target cell types. It is generally considered a lymphotropic virus due to its etiologic role in infectious mononucleosis, its close association with Burkitt's lymphoma and to the ease with which it can infect B lymphocytes in vitro (9-11). The presence of EBNA and EBV-DNA in nasopharyngeal carcinoma - an epithelial malignancy - makes it clear that EBV can infect epithelial tissues. In the tumors, as well as in the peripheral blood lymphocytes from acute IM patients, the virus transforms the cells and becomes latent. Although the viral genome and its expression can be readily demonstrated by DNA hybridization and EBNA immunofluorescence, electron-microscopy on the tissues have been uniformly negative (12-16). In the infected tumors and B lymphocytes, no active viral replication occurs after the transformation event. BL tumor derived cell lines and a small number of lymphoblastoid lines can be induced to enter a productive viral infection cycle, but usually not without laboratory manipulations. While it is possible, latently infected B lymphocytes are unlikely to be the reservoirs for EB infectious viruses. EBV replication in peripheral blood lymphocytes appear to be under stringent host regulations both in vivo and in vitro. Yet, copious amounts of extra-cellular virus can be found in the saliva of acute IM patients and patients showing immunosuppression (17,18). The source of the infectious viruses in these conditions remains and enigma.

Recent attempts to identify a possible reservoir in the oropharynx have yielded interesting results. Work by Sixeby and colleagues showed that both EBV-DNA and transcript RNA can be demonstrated in desquamated epithelial cells recovered from the oropharynx of IM patients (19). The presence of EBV-DNA in the nuclei of these cells clearly indicated their susceptibility to the virus. Although structural components such as VCA or complete virus particles were not demonstrated in the report, the presence of EBV-specific RNA was consistent with viral expression. The source of the desquamated cells is not yet known. More recently, Wolf and colleagues (20) have used in-situ hybridization and reassociation kinetics to establish the presence of EBV genomes in 3 post-mortem or operative specimens of parotid gland. Again, EM evidence of virus particles and immunofluorescence described.

From our study of oral hairy leukoplakia lesions, we now have strong evidence that EBV can and does replicate in the epithelial cells of the tongue. The infection is fully permissive with large number of viral particles both in the nuclei and cytoplasm of the infected cells, as seen in the thin sections. Immunofluorescence staining of the lesions with reference specific sera identified the herpes-like virus to be EBV and not HSV, VZV or CMV. The EB virus is associated with lesions only. Healthy buccal mucosa from the same patients were negative.

Evidence for the coexistence of papilloma virus with EB virus in the same cell type is the single most intriguing observation of the study. Hairy leukoplakia may provide an opportunity to explain and study another facet of EBV pathogenesis. In our HL series, 71% of the bipsies contained papillomavirus antigen. Using EBV-specific immunostaining, most specimens examined for both viruses were positive for both viruses. In a single case in which only papillomavirus was evident, the patient's anti-EBV VCA titers were unusually low (1:320), suggesting that the negative EBV results on the tissue were not a case of sampling error. To date, no HL lesions contained EBV only.

These findings suggest several intriguing possibilities. First, that the coexistence of the two viruses is not fortuitous. Second, infections of any one cell by the two may occur successively, e.g., papillomavirus may induce the required EBV receptors on the cells, facilitating the latters' entry and subsequent replication. In vitro transplantation of EBV membrane receptors have not demonstrated that the human epithelium lacked the necessary receptors, but not the necessary machinery for viral replications (21). At the same time, there are also in vitro data to suggest that active EBV replication occurs in these cells during terminal differentiation(22). Our observations appear to be an in vivo counterpart to the in vitro situation. Papillomavirus replication is also known to occur only in terminally differentiating cells.

The limited quantity of any single biopsy did not permit viral cultures except in a very small number of patients. Preliminary attempts have yielded negative results for HSV, VZV and CMV. We are also attempting cultivation of EBV. The relationship between HL and AIDS associated retroviruses is currently under investigation.

REFERENCES

1. M. A. Karnovsky, A formaldehyde-glutaraldehyde fixative of high osmolarity for use in electron microscopy, J. Cell Biol. 27:137A-138A (1965).
2. W. Henle, G. Henle, and C. A. Horowitz, Infectious mononucleosis and Epstein-Barr virus associated malignancies, in: "Diagnostic Procedures for Viral, Rickettsial and Chlamydial Infections," E. H. Lennette, N. J. Schmidt, eds. 5th edition, American Public Health Association Washington, D. C. (1979).
3. B. M. Reedman, G. Klein, Cellular localizaton of an Epstein-Barr virus (EBV)-associated complement-fixing antigen in producer and non-producer lymphoblastoid cell lines, Int. J. Cancer 11:499-520 (1973).
4. J. L. Zeigler, W. L. Drew, R. C. Miner et al., Outbreak of Burkitt's like lymphoma in homosexual men, The Lancet, Sept. 18:631-633 (1982).
5. Centers for Disease Control, Acquired immunodeficiency syndrome (AIDS) update - United States, MMWR 32:309-11 (1983).
6. A. E. Dunn and M. M. Ogilvie, Intranuclear virus particles in human genital wart tissue: Observations on the ultrastructure of the epidermal layer, J. Ultrastruc. Res. 22:282-295 (1968).
7. J. D. Oriel and J. D. Almeida, Demonstration of virus particles in human genital warts, Brit. J. vener Dis. 46:37 (1970).
8. M. G. Williams, A. F. Howatson, J. D. Almeida, Morphological characterization of the virus of the human common wart (verruca vulgaris), Nature 189:895-897 (1961).
9. G. Henle and W. Henle, The virus as the etiologic agent of infectious mononucleosis, in "The Epstein-Barr Virus," M. A. Epstein and B. G. Achong, eds., Springer Verlag, Berlin, Heidelberg, New York (1979).
10. H. zurHausen, H. Schulte-Holtausen, G. Klein et al., EBV DNA in biopsies of Burkitt's tumors and anaplastic carcinomas of the nasopharynx, Nature 228:1056-1058 (1970).
11. V. Diehl, G. Henle, W. Henle et al., Demonstration of a herpes group virus in cultures of peripheral leukocytes from patients with infectious mononucleosis, J. Virol. 2:663-669 (1968).

12. M. Nonoyama, C. H. Huang, J. S. Pagano et al., DNA of Epstein-Barr virus detected in tissue of Burkitt's lymphoma and nasopharyngeal carcinoma, Proc. Nat. Acad. Sci., 70:3265-3268 (1973).
13. T. Lindahl, G. Klein, B. Johansson et al., Relationship between Epstein-Barr virus (EBV) DNA and the determined nuclear antigen (EBNA) in Burkitt lymphoma biopsies and other lymphoproliferative diseases, Int. J. Cancer 13:764-722 (1974).
14. M. A. Epstein, B. G. Achong, Y. M. Barr, Virus particles in cultured lymphoblasts from Burkitt's lymphoma, The Lancet 702-703 (1964).
15. J. S. Nadkarmi, J. J. Nadkarmi et al., Epstein-Barr viral antigens in Burkitt Tumor biopsies and early cultures, Int. J. Cancer 6:10-17 (1970).
16. L. Gassolo, G. de The, M. Vuillaume et al., Nasopharyngeal carcinoma II, Ultrastructure of normal mucosa, tumor biopsies and subsequent epithelial growth in vivo, J. Nat. Cancer Inst. 48:73-86 (1972).
17. G. Miller, J. C. Niederman and L. Andrews, Prolonged oropharyngeal excretion of Epstein-Barr virus following infectious mononucleosis, N. Eng. J. Med. 137:140-147 (1973).
18. S. H. Cheeseman, W. Henle, R. H. Rubin et al., Epstein-Barr virus infection in Renal Transplants, Ann. of Int. Med. 93:39-42 (1980).
19. J. W. Sixbey, J. G. Nedrud, N. Raab-Traub et al., Epstein-Barr virus replication in oropharyngeal epithelial cells, N. Eng. J. Med. 310:1225-1230 (1984).
20. H. Wolf, G. J. Bayliss, E. Wilmes, Biologic properties of Epstein-Barr virus, in: "Nasopharyngeal Carcinoma," Cancer Campaign, Vol. 15, E. Grundman G. R. F. Krueger, and D. V. Ablashi eds., Stuttgart: Fisher-Verlag (1981).
21. I. M. Shapiro, D. J. Volsky, Infection of normal human epithelial cells by Epstein-Barr virus, Science 219:1225-1228 (1983).
22. J. W. Sixbey, E. H. Vesterinen, J. G. Nedral et al., Replication of Epstein-Barr virus in human epithelial cells infected in vitro., Nature 306:480-483 (1983).

THYMOSIN IN THE STAGING AND TREATMENT OF HLTV-III POSITIVE HOMOSEXUALS AND HEMOPHILIACS WITH AIDS-RELATED IMMUNE DYSFUNCTION

Allan L. Goldstein, Paul H. Naylor, Richard S. Schulof,
Gary L. Simon, Marcelo B. Sztein, and Craig M. Kessler,
Majorie Robert-Guroff, and Robert C. Gallo*
The George Washington Univ. Medical Ctr., Wash., D.C. 20037
National Cancer Institute*, Bethesda, MD 20205

INTRODUCTION

The paralysis and destruction of the thymic dependent immune system has become the hallmark of the acquired immune deficiency syndrome (AIDS) (1). Clinical symptoms of the disease usually include a progressive decline in essentially all thymus mediated immune functions, an increase in susceptibility to pneumocystis carinii pneumonia and other opportunistic infections, and an increase in the incidence of Kaposi's sarcoma and a number of lymphoid tumors (2-4). The current prognosis for patients with AIDS is dismal. Over 7,000 cases of AIDS have now been reported to the Center for Disease Control and over 70% of the patients have died. Immunological abnormalities which accompany the disease include a decline in helper T-cell number and function, a decline in lymphocyte reactivity to mitogens and antigens, decreased production of lymphokines (such as T-cell growth factor, IL-2, and interferon), and an increase in thymosin α_1 like cross-reacting material in serum. The presence of antibodies to a number of viruses has been documented and a recently described retrovirus designated as HTLV-III has been implicated as the cause of AIDS (1,5,6). To date AIDS has been confined primarily to individuals who fall into a relatively small number of risk groups. They include homosexuals (78 %), IV drug addicts (14 %), Haitians (3 %), and hemophiliacs (1 %) (1). The remaining small number of individuals (4 %) are generally found to be associated in some way with the defined risk groups.

Recent studies have found that many of the individuals in the risk groups have some degree of AIDS-like immune dysfunction (2-4). These abnormalities are manifested as lymphadenopathy, low helper-to-suppressor T-cell ratios, impaired T-cell responsiveness, elevated serum levels of thymosin α_1 , increased evidence of previous multiple viral infections (eg. HTLV-III, EBV, CMV, etc) as well as changes in a variety of other "surrogate markers". However, since these risk groups do not have AIDS associated diseases such as Kaposi's Sarcoma or pneumocystis carinii, there is currently no adequate classification of their syndrome. It is estimated that only about 10% of the at risk groups which are HTLV-III positive will progress to AIDS within two or three years of their diagnosis and during the interim these individuals will manifest increasing severe immune deficiencies and opportunistic infections (7,8). To date, it is still not possible to predict with certainty which individual members of the risk groups who will develop frank AIDS. The development of a diagnostic test(s) to help distinguish between exposure to HTLV-III and those destined to progress to frank AIDS will be of considerable value to the clinician in designing meaningful treatment strategies for pre-AIDS patients.

Our research efforts have focused on two of the relatively high risk populations, homosexuals and hemophiliacs, and are centered around our hypothesis that the thymus plays a pivotal role in AIDS (1,4).

Our first goal is the identification of the mechanism and events which result in abnormally high levels of thymosin α_1 (or thymosin α_1 like cross-reactivity) in the serum of individuals despite their immune depression and the presence of a lymphotrophic retrovirus (HTLV-III). These studies may help to separate those individuals that have been exposed to HTLV-III from the smaller group of individuals who will eventually progress to AIDS.

Our second goal is a therapeutic approach using thymosin as an immune modulator in patients at risk for developing AIDS in an attempt to prevent or reverse the decline in T-cell mediated immunity which is prevalent in the homosexual/hemophiliac populations. Preliminary results indicate that thymic hormones may be useful in the diagnosis of AIDS and may provide a means to improve the immune status of high risk populations.

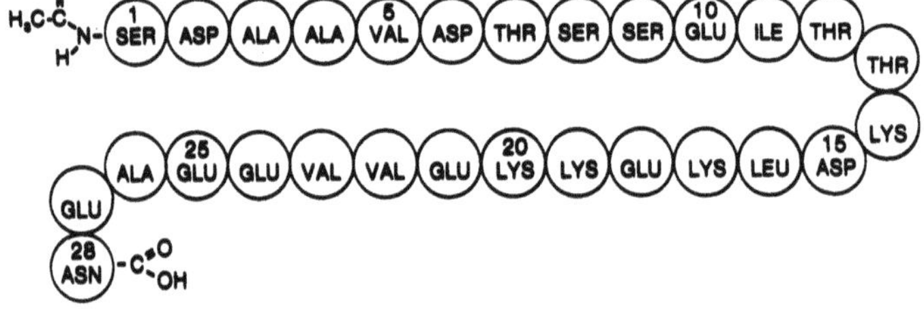

Figure 1. Amino Acid Sequence of Thymosin α_1.

Thymosin α_1

Thymosin fraction 5 (TF-5) is a partially purified thymic preparation which is effective in restoring immunological reactivity in many instances of immunodeficiency and/or suppression (9,10). Thymosin α_1 as shown in Figure 1, is a 28 amino acid peptide which was first isolated from TF-5 and has many of the immunological activities of TF-5 (9,10,11)

Our studies on the chemistry and biology of thymosins indicates that the peptides in TF-5 consist of three groups of biological active molecules. These are: 1) hormones produced in thymic epithelial cells such as thymosin α_1 which circulate in the blood and control a number of physiological processes; 2) lymphokine-like molecules isolated from thymocytes and; 3) non-specific peptides that is, nonspecific peptides brought through the isolation procedures.

There is also a substantial body of evidence that the partially purified TF-5 is active in all three major compartments of the lymphoid system (bone marrow, thymus and peripheral lymphoid tissues) in influencing the maturation, differentiation and activation of T-cells. The purified peptides appear, however, to have selective sites of action and, to date, none of the isolated peptides contains the complete spectrum of biological activity identified for TF-5. These results have led to the hypothesis that T-cell differentiation, maturation and activation require multiple steps and multiple peptides (9,10). It also follows that sequential synergistic effects might occur with TF-5 that could only be mimicked by a combination of purified peptides.

Recent histochemical and immunofluorescence studies (using the same anti- α_1 antibody prepared for the thymosin α_1 radioimmunoassay) have documented the localization of thymosin α_1-producing cells primarily to the epithelial cells of the thymus medulla but also to a lesser degree within the ring of subcapsular cortical surface epithelial cells (12). Immunofluorescence studies indicate that thymosin α_1 is not present in thymocytes nor in spleen sections but are present on the surface of a small number ($< 1\%$) of peripheral blood lymphocytes (13).

Using a cell-free wheat germ system to assess the translation of messenger RNA from calf thymus, it has been demonstrated that the radioactive products are immunoprecipitable with antisera against thymosin α_1 and the isolated peptide products are identical to those expected from tryptic peptides from thymosin α_1 (14). Low et al., have also demonstrated (using HPLC and RIA methodologies) that thymosin α_1 is present in thymus extracted with saline but not guanidine-hydrochloride (15). Thus, these results suggest that not only is thymosin α_1 synthesized in the thymus but it is synthesized as a larger molecular weight precursor. In more recent studies, it has been shown that a polypeptide in the thymus containing 112 amino acid residues (M.W. 12,000 Daltons) with the thymosin α_1 sequence at its NH_2-terminus, may be the prohormone from which thymosin α_1 and other fragments are generated during extraction procedures (16).The biological activities of TF-5 and thymosin α_1 have been extensively investigated and compared. Thymosin α_1 influences not only immature precursor cells but thymocytes and peripheral blood lymphocytes. These observations are consistant with its localization within the thymus as well as its circulation in serum. In vivo, thymosin α_1 has been shown to increase helper T-cell function and to improve survival of patients following treatment of non-oat cell lung cancers with radiotherapy (17).

Thymosin α_1 in serum

Using a radioimmunoassay (RIA) for thymosin α_1 developed in our laboratory, we have documented the presence of thymosin α_1 in human blood (18). There is a high degree of homology and immunological cross-reactivity in all species of thymosin α_1 examined by RIA and HPLC (15). Thymosin α_1 in adult serum is bound to a carrier protein of

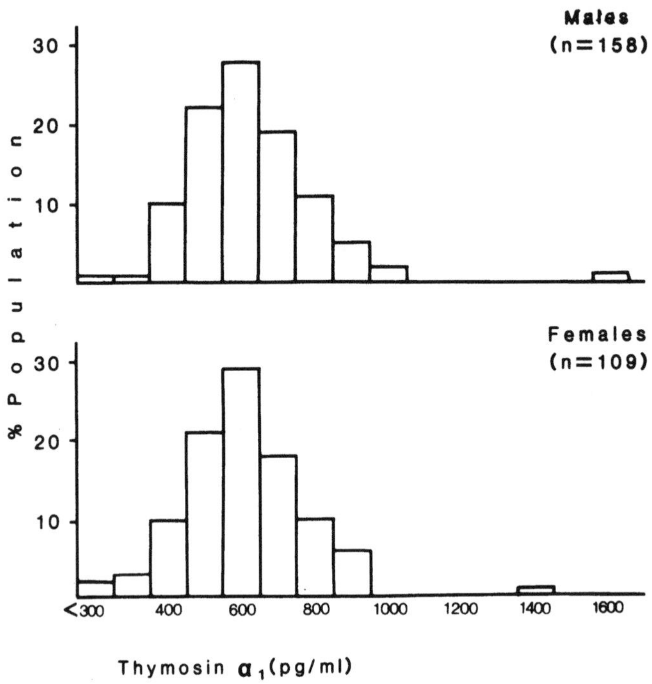

Figure 2. Thymosin α_1 levels in the serum from normal Red Cross Blood Donors.

molecular weight > 25,000 daltons (19). In man, thymosin α_1 concentrations are highest in the fetal circulation and decrease rapidly after birth (18). In adults, thymosin α_1 levels are rarely (< 1%) above 992 pg/ml. This value is 2 standard deviations from the mean of 265 Red Cross volunteer donors from the Washington, D.C. area (mean ± S.D. = 664 ± 164). Both males and females and individuals between the ages of 20 and 50 were included in this study (Fig 2).

We have recently identified several groups of "patients" whose levels of thymosin α_1 are not within this normal range (1,3,4,20-23). Lower than normal levels have been found in the blood of children with primary immunodeficiency diseases, such as DiGeorge Syndrome and a variety of other thymic hypoplasias associated with decreased helper T-cells, lymphopenia and immune dysfunction (4). Higher than normal values (> 2 standard deviations from the mean) have been reported in adults and children with AIDS (Figure 3), certain homosexuals (Figure 3), certain hemophiliacs (21,22) and individuals with some types of T-cell leukemia (1).

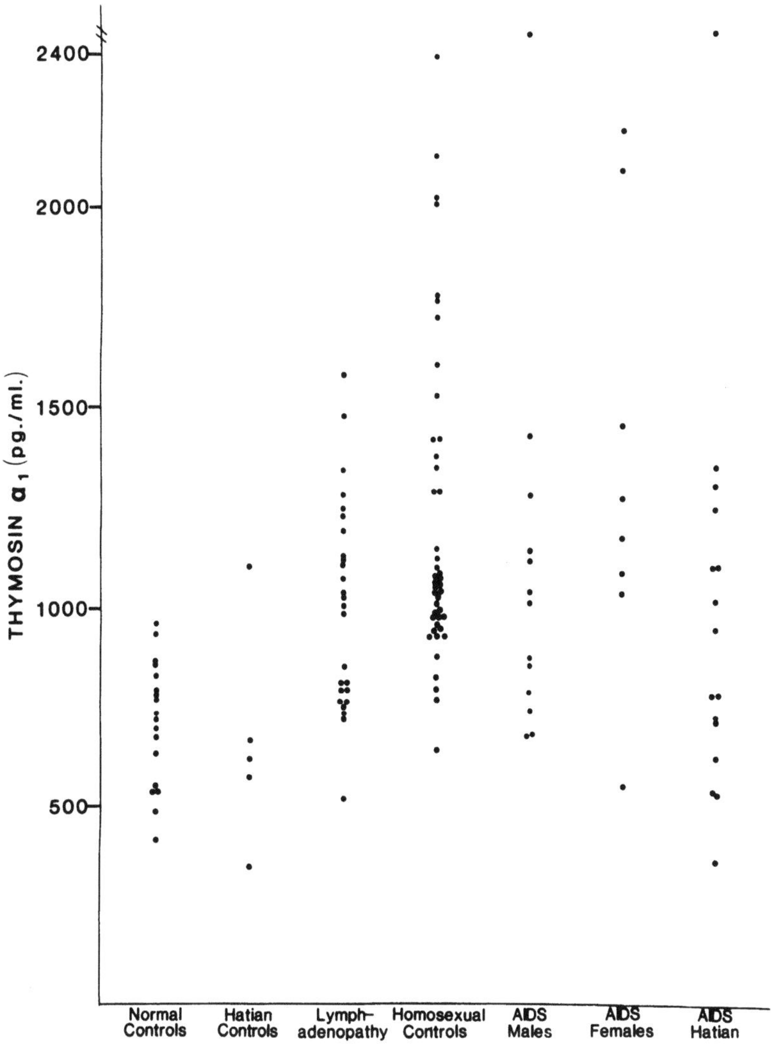

Figure 3. Thymosin α_1 levels in serum from patients with AIDS or at risk for AIDS. Serum provided by Dr. Thomas Spira, Centers for Disease Control.

Hypothesis

While the abnormally low levels in immune deficiencies are readily explained, the reason for elevated level has not been clearly defined. At least three hypotheses for the elevated levels of thymosin α_1 would explain these results (Figure 4). One possibility is that we are looking at end organ failure in the presence of an elevated level of biologically active peptides. In this case, abnormal (i.e. virus infected) lymphocytes would not respond and the result would be breakdown of normal feedback channels. A second possibility is that the elevated levels are due to cross-reactive proteins which are not identical to the biological active material. The source of this material could be a viral infected thymus and/or lymphocytes. A third hypothesis is the ectopic production of thymosin α_1. Such a possibility is raised by the observation that HTLV-III virus can be found in many tissues (including brain) and the fact that certain areas of the brain are known to have high levels of thymosin α_1(9,12). The elevated levels of thymosin α_1 could tip the delicate balance of the immune system and result in an increase in suppressor or decrease in helper cells.

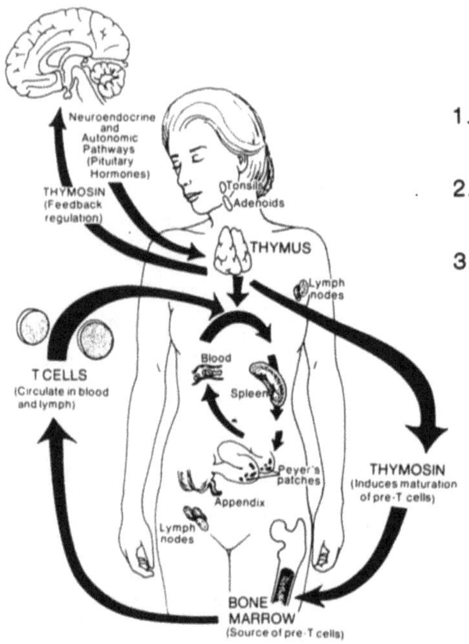

1. END ORGAN FAILURE

2. THYMUS MALFUNCTION

3. ECTOPIC PRODUCTION

Figure 4. Proposed mechanisms for elevated thymosin α_1 in AIDS.

High Pressure Liquid Chromatography (HPLC) Analysis of Thymosin α_1 in Serum.

We have demonstrated that normal serum contains authentic thymosin α_1 identical to the hormone isolated from thymus tissue by the following criterion: 1) an antibody raised to synthetic thymosin α_1 and specific for thymosin α_1 can be used to measure serum levels of thymosin α_1 via RIA (18); 2) an affinity column prepared using anti-thymosin α_1 antibodies will extract a form of thymosin α_1 from Cohn IV-I fractionated human plasma (24) which has an identical HPLC retention time and isoelectric focusing profile to natural and synthetic thymosin α_1 , and 3) using a C18 SEP-PAK elution, followed by high performance liquid chromatography on a C18 μBondapak column (under reverse phase conditions) a peak which cross-reacts with the anti-thymosin α_1 antibody and has a retention time identical to thymosin α_1 can be demonstrated (Figure 5) (25).

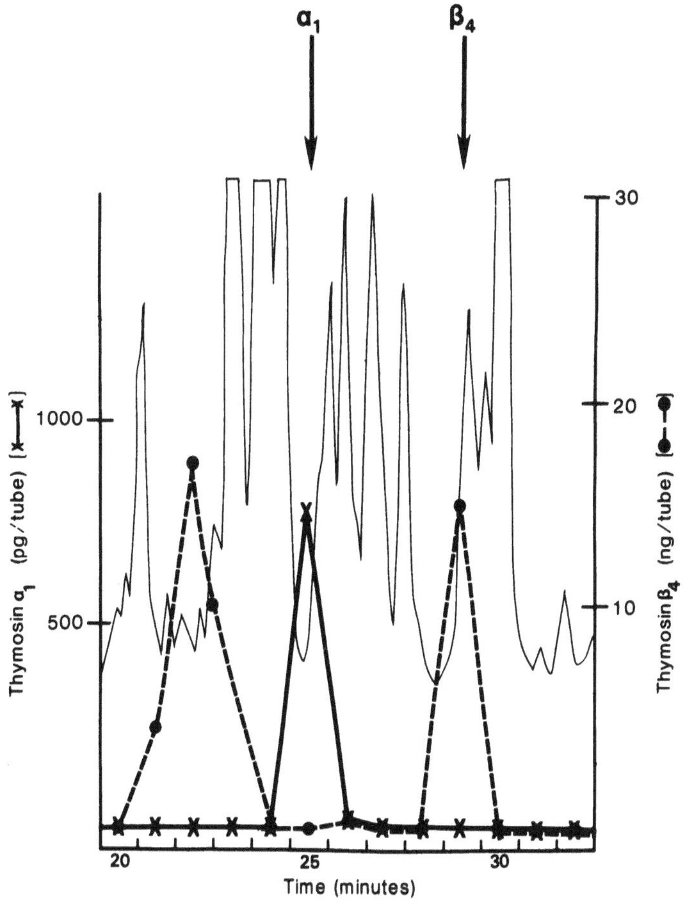

Figure 5. Human serum subjected to high performance liquid chromatography and eluted samples assayed for thymosin α_1 and thymosin β_4.

Using SEP-PAK concentration, HPLC elution, and RIA detection, we have evaluated serum from several homosexuals. To date, two different profiles have been seen (Figure 6). In one group (panel B), the profile is similar to that of a pool of normal donors. In the other group (Panel C), there is essentially, no detectable thymosin α_1. We are currently expanding the number of samples of both normals and homosexuals to further define these observations. If there are two readily distinguishable groups of at risk homosexuals, one with normal thymosin α_1 levels and the other with deficient levels of authentic thymosin α_1 then this could have important implications for developing therapy protocols. The results to date are interesting in that a large number of the homosexuals have had elevated levels of a serum substance, that cross-reacts with an antibody to thymosin α_1 by RIA, yet appears to have little or no authentic thymosin α_1 when analyzed by HPLC. We are attempting to identify the cross-reactive, non-authentic material since it clearly is not in the 20-30 minute retention time region of the HPLC profile from which we collect thymosin α_1 samples for RIA analysis. It is also not yet possible to quantitate accurately the cross-reactivity of thymosin α_1 in the peaks in which levels of thymosin α_1 can be measured and to compare them to the levels in normal serum. Such a quantitative comparison may prove useful, since a decline in authentic thymosin α_1 below a "normal" range may be a more accurate measure of AIDS risk than an increase in non-authentic cross-reactive thymosin α_1.

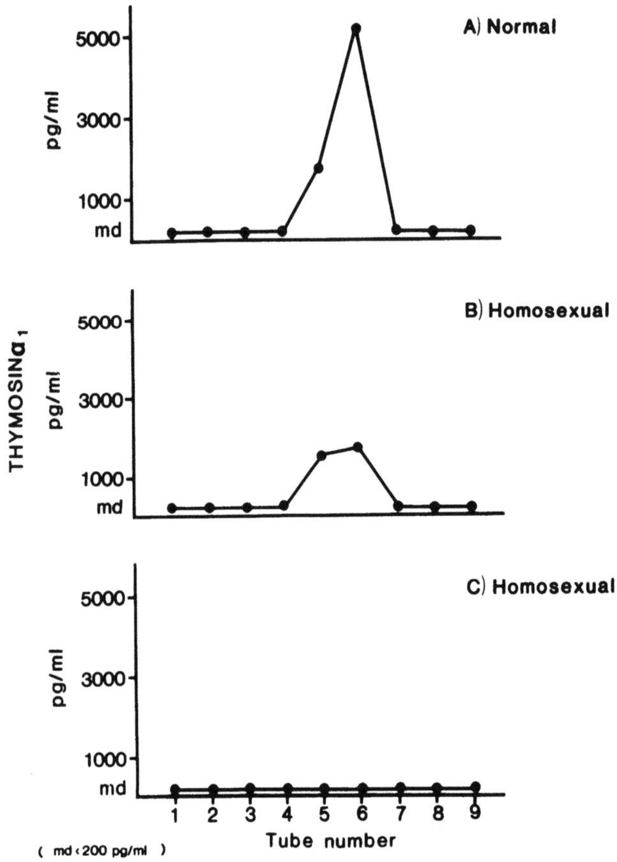

Figure 6. Serum from normal and homosexual donors subjected to high performance liquid chromotography and eluted samples assayed for thymosin α_1.

Serum Thymosin α_1 and HTLV-III.

In the studies to date, the immunoreactive thymosin α_1 levels in serum of patients with AIDS, homosexuals and hemophiliacs have not always correlated with a decrease in helper/suppressor T-cell ratios (3,20). We have now determined that the presence of antibodies to HTLV-III do not usually correlate with elevated levels of thymosin α_1. (Table 1). In many respects, this is encouraging if thymosin α_1 levels are to be useful indicators of real risk for AIDS since only about 10% of patients with HTLV-III antibodies progress to frank AIDS over a one year period. We have not yet attempted to correlate the presence of "authentic thymosin α_1 to any other AIDS markers.

TABLE 1
Immune Parameters in Homosexuals (HO) and Hemopheliacs (HE) at risk for AIDS.

Patients	Age (yrs)	H/S	HTLV-III*	Thymosin α_1 (pg/ml)
HO	33	1.7	+	705
HO	33	1.2	+	493
HO	26	0.9	+	1055
HO	28	0.8	+	580
HO	35	0.7	+	1106
HO	37	0.5	+	932
HO	51	0.2	+	1072
HO	39	0.1	+	324
HO	52	1.2	-	1217
HO	36	.7	-	633
HO	34	.5	-	867
HE/HO	24	.6	+	1016
HE	24	1.1	+	733
HE	27	.6	+	746
HE	36	.5	+	502

* By Elisa and Western Blot Assays

Thymosin Fraction 5 Treatment in Homosexuals and Hemophiliacs At Risk for AIDS

We have initiated a pilot study to evaluate the efficacy of TF-5 administration in homosexuals and hemophiliacs (4). We elected to study patients in "at risk" groups with immune dysfunction because of our belief that once frank AIDS develops, there is less likelihood that non-specific biological response modifiers will alter the progression of the disease.

In this study, at the George Washington University Medical Center, we have been evaluating both the in vitro and in vivo immunorestorative action of TF-5 in subjects defined by us as at risk for developing AIDS. Candidates in this trial must be immunosuppressed (low T4:T8 ratios) male homosexuals or hemophiliacs without frank AIDS, that is, without a prior history of opportunistic infections or an AIDS-associated malignancy. In our laboratory, the normal mean OKT4/OKT8 T-cell ratio in normal subjects is 2.0 ± 0.8 S.D. We consider someone as eligible for our pilot trial if he exhibits an appropriate risk factor and an OKT4/OKT8 ratio of more than one standard deviation below the normal mean (i.e. < 1.2) on each of 3 successive monthly testings. Subsequent, analysis of HTLV-III has indicated that almost all were also positive for antibody to the virus. To date 32 patients have been entered and have been treated with either 30 mg (10 patients), 60 mg (10 patients), or 120 mg (12 patients) of TF-5 by daily SQ injection for 10 weeks. Thymosin treatment has been well tolerated with the only side effect being erythema and pain at the injection site requiring termination of treatment in three of the patients. The results of the trial are currently being analyzed and only preliminary data will be presented here. As shown in Figure 7, four of the five initial subjects (60 mg treatment group) studied had an improvement in their PHA-induced production of IL-2 response and two with depressed MLR's responded with an increase in their MLR values. Serum thymosin α_1 levels were found to also increase following treatment. The functional immune improvement following administration of thymosin may be another indicator that the elevated levels of thymosin α_1 in some of these individuals may not be biologically active. We are currently completing the evaluation of 12 patients that received a higher (120 mg/day) dose and 10 patients that received a lower (30 mg/day) dose of TF-5. Preliminary analysis of these studies suggest that the 60 mg per day is the optimal dose for restoration of some functional immune responses.

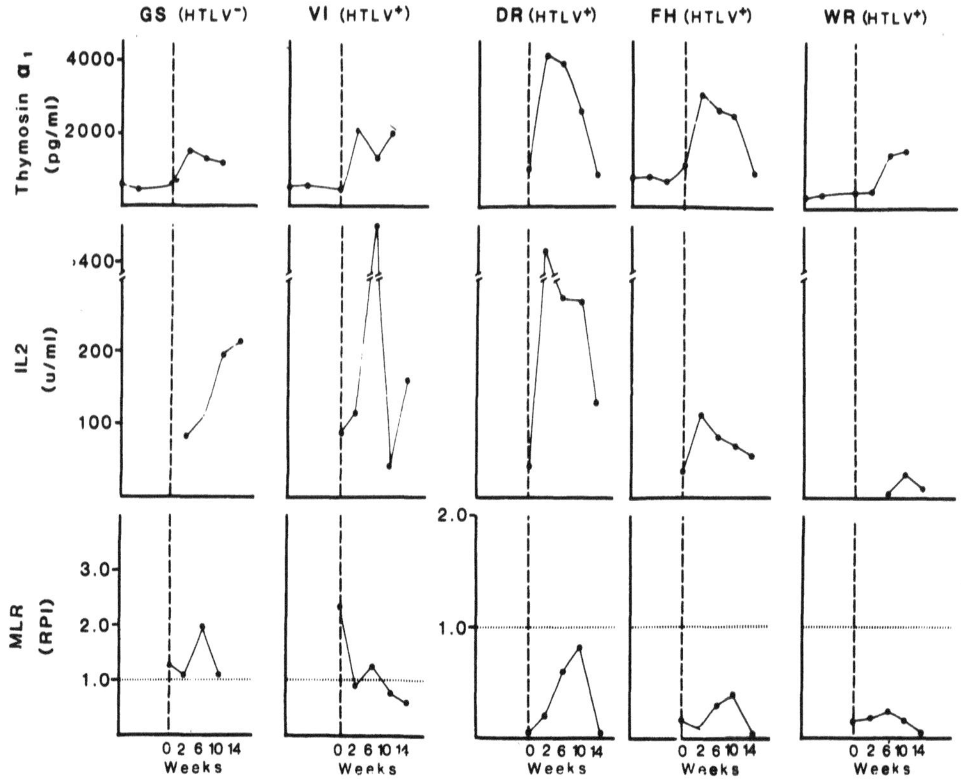

Figure 7. Changes in thymosin α_1, PHA-induced interleukin-2 production and mixed lymphocyte reactivity in homosexuals treated daily with TF-5 (60 mg).

CONCLUSIONS

Individuals with AIDS have a more severe form of thymus-mediated immune dysfunction and immune paralysis than homosexuals and hemophiliacs "at risk" for AIDS. Recently, a number of studies have indicated a wide spread exposure of hemophiliacs and homosexuals to HTLV-III, the virus implicated in AIDS. Individuals with AIDS also have abnormal thymus morphology, abnormally low levels of thymic hormone activity (thymulin) as measured by bioassay and an abnormally elevated level of thymosin α_1 as measured by RIA. Many homosexuals and hemophiliacs at risk for AIDS also have elevated levels of thymosin α_1 but the elevated levels do not appear to correlate with parameters such as HTLV-III antibody titers or helper/suppressor T-cell ratios. Administration of TF-5 results in increases in serum thymosin α_1 and improves specific immune functions (MLR and IL-2) in homosexuals and hemophiliacs with low T4/T8 ratios most of which are HTLV-III positive.

The results of our studies suggest: 1) evaluating authentic thymosin α_1 in the blood may be of help in distinguishing between the larger group of individuals that are HTLV-III positive from the smaller group of individuals that are destined to develop AIDS; 2) TF-5 may modulate AIDS-like immune dysfunction by increasing levels of biologically active thymosin α_1 and 3) early intervention with thymosin or other thymomimetic agents in individuals at risk for AIDS may be beneficial in preventing the later progression to AIDS.

Finally, if our preliminary studies are correct, and HTLV-III positive individuals who have authentic and non-authentic serum thymosin α_1 can be identified and followed longitudinally such an evaluation may provide an indication of the chances of individuals at risk to progress to AIDS. Such studies would help to identify candidates for early intervention with thymosin or other thymomimetic agents.

Acknowledgements

These studies are supported in part by grants and/or gifts from the NIH (CA24974), Alpha One Biomedicals, Inc. and Hoffmann-La Roche, Inc.

REFERENCES

1. Naylor, P.H. and Goldstein, A.L. 1984. Bioessays 1, 63.
2. CDC Task Force, 1984, M.M.W.R., 33, 589.
3. Hersh, E.M., Reuben, J.M., Rios, A., Newell, G.R., Mansell, P.W., McClure, J.E. and Goldstein, A.L. 1983. N. Engl. J. Med. 308, 45.
4. Naylor, P.H., Schulof, R.S., Sztein, M.B., Spira, T.J., McCurdy, P.R., Kessler, C.M., Simon, G., and Goldstein, A.L., N.Y.A.S. Monograph on AIDS (in press).
5. Popovic, M., Sarngadharan, M.G., Read, E. & Gallo, R.C. 1984. Science, 244, 497.
6. Vilmer, E., Rouzioux, C., Vezinet-Brun, F., Fischer, A., Chermann, J.C., Barre-Sinoussi, F., Gazengel, C., Dauguet, C., Manigne, P., Griscelli, C. and Motangnier, L. 1984. Lancet i, 753.
7. Mather-Wagh, U., Enlow, R.W., Spegland, I., et al., 1984, Lancet 1, 1033.
8. Abrams, D.I., Lewis, B.J., Beckstead, J.H., Casavant, C.A., and Drew, W.L., 1984, Ann. Intern. Med., 100, 801.
9. Goldstein, A.L., T.L.K. Low, M.M. Zatz, N.R. Hall, P.H. Naylor. 1983. Clin. in Immunol. and Allergy 3, 119.

10. Schulof, R.S. and A.L. Goldstein. 1983. Rec. Adv. in Clin. Immunol. 3. 243.
11. Goldstein, A.L., Low, T.L.K., McAdoo, M., McClure, J., Thurman, G.B., Rossio, J., Lai, C-Y., Chang, D., Wong, S.S., Harvey, C., Ramel, A.H. and Meinhofer, J. 1977. Proc. Nat. Acad. Sci. USA 74, 725.
12. Goldstein, A.L., T.L.K. Low, G.B. Thurman, M. Zatz, N.R. Hall, J. Chen, S-K. Hu, P.B. Naylor and J.E. McClure. 1981. Rec. Prog. Hormone Res. 37,369.
13. Dalakas, M.C., Rose, J.W., Paul, J., Engel, W.K., McClure, J.E. and Goldstein, A.L. 1983. Neurology 33, 144.
14. Freire, M., Hannappel, E., Rey, M., Freire, S.M., Kide, H. and Horecker, B.L. 1981. Proc. Natl. Acad. Sci. 78, 192.
15. Low, T.L.K., McClure, J.E., Spangelo, B.L., Low, T.L.K. and Goldstein, A.L. 1983. J. Chromatography 266, 533.
16. Haritos, A.A., Goodall, G.J. and Horecker, B.L., 1984, Proc. Natl. Sci., USA, 81, 1008-1011.
17. Schulof, R.S., Lloyd, M., Cox, J., Palazynski, S.R., McClure, J.E., Incefy, G.S. and and Goldstein, A.L. IN: Thymic Hormones and Lymphokines (A.L. Goldstein, ed.), 601.
18. McClure, J.E., Lameris, N., Wara, D.W. and Goldstein, A.L. 1982. J. Immunol. 128, 368.
19. Naylor, P.H., Spangelo, B.L., Low, T.L.K. and Goldstein, A.L. 1983. 65th Annual Meeting of the Endocrine Society #184.
20. Biggar, R.J., Naylor, P.H., Goldstein, A.L., Melby, M.,Mannovil, D.L., Strong, D.M. 1983. N. Engl. J.Med. 309, 49.
21. Kreiss, J.K., Lawrence, D.N., Kasper, C.K., Goldstein, A.L., Naylor, P.H., McLane, M.F., Lee, T-H., Essex, M., 1984. Annals Int. Med. 100, 178.
22. Kessler, C.M., Schulof, R.S., Goldstein, A.L., Naylor, P.H., Phillips, T.M., Luban, N.L.C., Kelleher, J.F. and Reaman, G.H. Brit. J. Hematology 1984, 58, 321.
23. Naylor, P.H. and Goldstein, A.L. 1983. Clin. Lett. 4, 126.

THE MECHANISM AND MODULATION OF IMMUNE DYSFUNCTION IN AIDS ASSOCIATED SYNDROMES

J. George Bekesi, Peter Tsang and Julia P. Roboz

Mount Sinai School of Medicine, Dept. Neoplastic Diseases
One Gustave L. Levy Place
New York, New York 10029

INTRODUCTION

Acquired immunodeficiency syndrome (AIDS) is an acute disease which is characterized by a profound dysfunction of cell mediated immunity including severe anergy,[1] marked reduction in the number of T-helper cells,[1,2,3,4,5] an apparent inversion of T-helper to T-suppressor cell ratio[2,4,5] and reduced natural killer cell function.[6,7,8,9] Most patients were reported to have increased levels of serum immunoglobulins.[3,4,6,7,8,10] Also, high titers of antibodies have been reported to cytomegalovirus (CMV), Epstein Barr Virus (EBV), and hepatitis virus.[11,12,13,14] The group considered to be at highest risk to develop AIDS are homosexual men some of whom are often promiscuous.[15]

Evidence for involvement of retroviruses in AIDS now appears certain. Three T-lymphotropic viruses: human T-cell leukemia virus HTLV III,[16,17,18] lymphadenopathy-associated viruses (LAV)[19,20] and immunodeficiency-associated virus (IDAV)[21] have been isolated from lymphocytes of individuals at risk and AIDS patients. It is conceivable that an accumulation of repeated assaults to their immune defenses by CMV, EBV, HTLV III/LAV, Herpes, hepatitis viruses, repeated semen exposures[15,21,22] and drug usage[1,2,23] may lead to irreversible immunodeficiencies and multiple infections in the final stages of this clinical syndrome.

Therapeutic approaches aimed to improve cell-mediated immunity (CMI) in homosexual males at risk and in AIDS patients have become the subject of intensive investigations. The effectiveness of a variety of biological and synthetic response modulators have been tested. Interferon, interleukin-2, and thymosine appeared to be equivocal as potentially useful biological modulators in AIDS and prodromal conditions.[5,6,7] Isoprinosine, the p-acetamidobenzoic acid salt of inosine dimethylamino-isopropanol, is an antiviral agent which has immuno-potentiating activities.[5,23,24,25,26,27,28,29] To obtain better understanding of the mode of its _in vitro_ action, the immune restorative effects of isoprinosine have been investigated on the functions of lymphocytes derived from male homosexuals with prodromal symptoms and AIDS patients. Results reported here are suggestive that isoprinosine has significant restorative influence on the lymphocyte function in individuals with prodromal symptoms.

TABLE 1.

LYMPHOCYTE SUBSETS IN HOMOSEXUALS AT RISK AND AIDS PATIENTS

STUDY SUBJECTS	PHENOTYPES+								
	Total T-Cells		Helper T-Cells		Suppressor T-Cells		T_h/T_s	Natural Killer Cells	
	%	Abs Nº	%	Abs Nº	%	Abs Nº		%	Abs Nº
CONTROL (heterosexual males)	69.7 ±18	1391 ±235	43.4 ±9	886 ±210	20.3 ±9	405 ±89	2.14	20.4 ±4.6	406 ±129
HOMOSEXUALS AT RISK DEVELOPING	58.8 ±16	1164 ±349	24.0* ±8	475* ±177	28.5 ±10	564 ±218	0.84*	21.8 ±5.1	431 ±243
AIDS PATIENTS	46.1* ±11	663* ±273	14.0 ±7	201* ±75	30.7 ±8	441 ±166	0.45*	15.7 ±3.2	226* ±111

+ Results are expressed as mean ± SD of percent and absolute number of indicated lymphocytes

* Student's "t" tests were computed between the control group and all other groups on phenotypic variables $p<.001$

Study Subjects

Three study groups were subjected to comprehensive clinical and immunological testings at Mount Sinai Medical Center in New York. 163 homosexual males at risk to develop AIDS (average age 34.7±7) with a mean leukocyte count of 5340±1092 mm^3 had general symptoms such as fever lasting more than 7 days, venereal and/or herpes infection, anogenital lesions weight loss greater than 10 lb.,diarrhea, and lymphadenopathy at multiple sites, all of which have been reported associated with acquired immune deficiency syndrome. Of the twenty-seven clinically diagnosed AIDS patients (average age 35.9±6) twenty-one were diagnosed with Kaposi's sarcoma and six with opportunistic infections. The third group was made up of 118 apparently healthy heterosexual males (average age: 43.3±8) with a mean leukocyte count of 6900±725.

Cell Surface Phenotypes

Examination of the following phenotype parameters: Total T, T-helper T-suppressor and NK-cells demonstrated significant aberrations within the group of 163 homosexual males and the 27 AIDS patients, but by different degrees. We observed reduction in the number of circulating T-lymphocytes and in the ratio of helper/suppressor T-lymphocytes (Table 1). The absolute number and the percentage of helper T-cells were markedly reduced in the homosexual population and to a higher degree in AIDS patients. Although homosexual males and AIDS patients showed higher percentage of T-suppressor cells compared to the heterosexual controls, no such pattern was apparent when the results were calculated on the basis of absolute numbers. Table 1 also depicts the lymphocyte subpopulation bearing Leu7 receptors specific for circulating NK-cells. The number of $Leu7^+$ cells were within the normal range both for control subjects and homosexual males at risk but were significantly reduced in the AIDS patients.

Lymphocyte Functions

The functional integrity of peripheral blood lymphocytes of the three study groups was assessed by means of lymphoblastogenesis with T-cell mitogen PHA and T-cell dependent B-lymphocyte mitogen PWM. Responses to both PHA and PWM were impaired in homosexuals at risk and to a greater degree in the AIDS groups. The magnitude of impaired lymphocyte function

Table 2. FUNCTIONAL INTEGRITY OF PBL

	T-Lymphocyte Function*	T-Cell Dependent B-Lymphocyte Function*
	c.p.m.	
Control (N=118) (heterosexual males)	99,540 ±18,610	97,620 ±19,710
High Risk Homosexual Males (N=163)	64,034** ±1,850	43,580** ±15,600
AIDS Patients (N=27)	28,768** ±16,000	17,300** ±14,000

* Results are expressed as mean c.p.m. ± SD

** Student "t" tests were computed between the control subjects values and all other groups (p <.001)

was consistent with the prodromal state among the homosexual males leading to more severe immunodepression in AIDS patients (see Table 2).

In summary, 30.1% of the homosexual subjects at risk showed deficiency in T-cell function, while 84.1% exhibited reduced T-cell dependent B-lymphocyte function. In comparison 96.3% of the 27 AIDS patients were deficient in lymphocyte functions.

The reduced pokeweed mitogen induced responses can be explained either by a reduction of T-helper cell associated functions or by increased T-suppressor cell action. When the absolute number of helper T-cells was plotted against PWM induced blastogenesis, 70.5% of the homosexual males and all AIDS patients values were as or below the 5th percentile of the heterosexual group for both parameters (Fig. 1) suggesting a close association of reduced helper T-cell number and B-lymphocyte dysfunction. Contrariwise response to T-cell dependent B cell mitogen response appeared to be unrelated to the number of suppressor T lymphocytes.

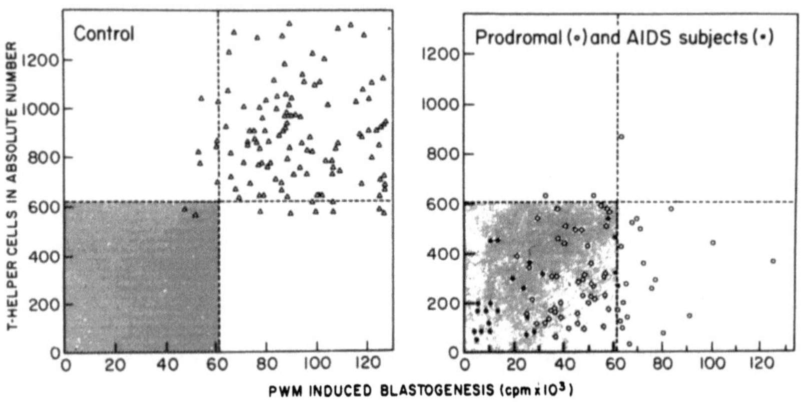

Figure 1. Association between the marked disease in helper T cell numbers and impaired response to PWM among prodromal homosexual males (o) and patients with AIDS (●). The shaded areas represent regions which contain the lower 5% of the matched control group of heterosexual males (Δ) with concurrent determinations on the respective parameters.

Suppressor T-Lymphocyte Subsets in AIDS

It has been suggested that in conjunction with a decrease in helper T-cell functions, elevated suppressor T-lymphocyte activity may also be a significant factor in the pathogenesis of AIDS. Although in the study presented above prodromal subjects and AIDS patients showed only in few cases slightly higher number of suppressor T-cells, compared to those of heterosexual control, no association was observed with altered lymphocyte functions. This lack of correlation does not rule out however, the possibility that a subset(s) of T-suppressor cells may be abnormally activated. Applying two color flow cytometric analysis and a panel of monoclonal antibodies that define functional subsets and stages of lymphocyte differentiation (Leu8, Leu15, HLA-DR) we examined the co-expression of these markers on the peripheral blood lymphocytes obtained from homosexual males at risk and AIDS patients with depressed B-cell function. Table 3 summarizes our findings.

TABLE 3.

CO-EXPRESSION OF SUPPRESSOR T-LYMPHOCYTES OF LEU2 WITH Ia, LEU8, LEU15 MONOCLONAL ANTIBODIES

STUDY SUBJECTS	SUPPRESSOR LYMPHOCYTE(Leu2) SUBSETS (%)+						Helper (Leu3) T-Lymphocytes Subset in (%)
	Activated Ts		Cytotoxic Ts		Precursor Ts	Effector Ts	
	2^+HLA-DR^+	2^+15^+	2^+HLA-DR^-	2^+15^-	2^+8^+	$2^+ 8^-$	
C O N T R O L (Heterosexual, males)	4.5 ± 1	4.5 ± 2	14.0 ± 5	13.3 ± 3	5.9 ± 2.8	10.8 ± 3	43.9 ± 9
Homosexuals at Risk	25.6* ± 5	13.0* ± 3	9.4 ± 5	20.3* ± 4	11.8* ± 3	20.8* ± 5	24.0 ± 8
AIDS PATIENTS	18.8* ± 3	14.1* ±1.8	5.0* ± 1	8.3 ± 6	7.7 ± 4	14.7 ± 3	14.0 ± 7

+ Results are expressed as mean ± SD of percent of the indicated lymphocyte subsets

* Student's "t" tests were computed between the control group and all other groups on phenotypic variables p=<.001

There was an overall increase in activated HLA-DR$^+$ lymphocytes with the elevation in T-suppressor Leu2$^+$ HLA-DR$^+$ cells representing the majority of the increase. An increase in suppressor precursor Leu2$^+$, Leu8$^+$, and effector Ts Leu2$^+$ Leu8$^-$ lymphocytes was detected in prodromal subjects. Our data also show an increase in the functionally active suppressor T-cells Leu2$^+$ Leu15$^+$ in both prodromal and AIDS patients whereas the reciprocal cytotoxic Ts-cells Leu2$^+$ Leu15$^-$ were elevated only in the high risk homosexual group. These results appear to demonstrate a possible defect in the feed back suppressor loop which regulates both the helper and suppressor T cell systems as well as B-cell functions prodromal subjects and in AIDS patients.

Modulation of Lymphocyte Functions by Isoprinosine

The clinical need for immunepotentiative agents to normalize altered immune functions led us to investigate a variety of biological modifiers including Isoprinosine (24)(26). Modulatory action of lymphokines on the NK-cell activity in prodromal subjects and AIDS patients was reported by us previously and will not be discussed in this report (6). In order to determine the possibility of normalizing the altered lymphocyte functions among prodromal homosexual males and AIDS patients using Isoprinosine, PHA and PWM induced blastic transformation was performed in the presence of this modulator.

Isoprinosine at 100 µg/ml was established to be optimal concentration in producing maximum modulation of lymphocytes derived from both normal and prodromal subjects. Among the heterosexual controls, incubation of PBL with optimum dose of isoprinosine resulted in a 25.4% increase in the PWM and 29.3% in the PHA induced lymphoblastogenesis (Table 4). A greater degree of increase in lymphocyte functions was achieved with isoprinosine, in both prodromal homosexuals and AIDS patients.

The mean increase in the PHA induced proliferation is 46.6% for the prodromal group and 45.8% of the AIDS group. Within this 79% of the prodromal subjects and none of the AIDS cases were actually normalized. In terms of the T-cell dependent B-cell function isoprinosine increased the prodromal subjects by 36.5% and the AIDS patients by 50%. Of this 63% of the prodromal subjects,none of the AIDS cases were again normalized. These observations appear to indicate the capacity of isoprinosine to restore at least partially the depressed cell mediated immunity associated with AIDS. However, complete normalization of the lymphocyte function is possible only at the prodromal stage although moderate improvement was observed in subjects with AIDS as well.

Conclusions:

Selected phenotypic and functional parameters have shown significant changes in prodromal homosexual males and patients with AIDS. Reduction in the number of circulating helper T-lymphocytes led to altered ratio of T-helper to T-suppressor subpopulations in both groups of subjects, although the number of T-suppressor cells remained comparable to the controls.

Responses to the T-cell mitogen (PHA) and the T-cell dependent B-cell mitogen (PWM) were impaired in prodromal subjects and to a higher degree in the AIDS group. The latter was associated with a significant reduction in the helper T-lymphocyte number but appeared unrelated to the suppressor T-lymphocytes. Further examination of the functional subsets of T-lymphocytes by a panel of monoclonal antibodies using two color flow cytometric techniques revealed that in both prodromal subjects and AIDS patients activated suppressor T-cells were elevated while reciprocal cytotoxic T-

TABLE 4.

MODULATION OF LYMPHOCYTE FUNCTION BY ISOPRINOSINE

STUDY GROUPS	LYMPHOCYTE TRANSFORMATION*					
	PHA -ISO	PHA +ISO	% Modulation	PWM -ISO	PWM +ISO	% Modulation[a]
	cpm x 1000			cpm x 1000		
CONTROL (Heterosexual, males)	96.3 ±19.5	123.5 ±22.0	29.3	92.6 ±21.5	116.2 ±23.1	25.4
Homosexuals at Risk	79.9 ±18.5	117.1 ±34.6	46.6	53.5 ±18.8	72.8 ±18.5	36.5
AIDS PATIENTS	28.8 ±17.3	41.5 ±28.3	45.8 ±15.9	17.3 ±24.9	26.0	50.0

* Results are expressed as mean ± SD of c.p.m. of incorporation of H^3TdR

(a) Percent of modulation by Isoprinosine = [(cpm + ISO - cpm - ISO)/cpm - ISO] x 100

suppressor cells (Leu2^{+} Leu15^{-} and Leu2^{+} HLA-DR^{-}) were significantly reduced. Both subsets of T-suppressor precursor and effector lymphocytes were elevated among the high risk homosexual males. These data suggest a defective regulatory control of helper and suppressor T-cells and the T-cell dependent B-lymphocyte function.

Immunomodulative action of Isoprinosine was tested in prodromal homosexual males and patients with AIDS where proliferative responses, particularly T-cell dependent B-cell function, were severely impaired. Co-cultivation of their lymphocytes with isoprinosine resulted in increase and in some cases, normalization, of lymphocyte functions as monitored by PHA, PW induced blastogenesis in the prodromal group. Similar degree of modulation, but never normalization of lymphocyte functions were noted in patients with AIDS. Based on this information the eventual prophylactic utilization of isoprinosine might be of value in prodromal homosexuals at high risk to develop AIDS.

Acknowledgment

This work was supported by the T.J. Martell Foundation for Cancer and Leukemia Research. The authors wish to acknowledge the technical assistance of Mrs. Khanitha Tangnavarad, Ms. Ratchanee Songsakphisarn and Mr. Mohammed Zanjani and the secretarial assistance of Ms. Diane Andujar.

REFERENCES

1. J. J. Goerdert, C. Y. Neuland, W. C. Wallen, M. H. Greene, D. L. Mann, C. Murray, D. M. Strong, J. F. Fraumeni, and W. A. Blattner, Amyl Nitrite May Alter T Lymphocytes in Homosexual Men, Lancet. 1:412 (1982).
2. J. M. Reuben, E. M. Hersh, P. W. Mansell, G. Newell, A. Rios, R. Rossen, A. L. Goldstein, and J. E. McClure, Immunological Characterization of Homosexual Males, Cancer Res. 43:897 (1983).
3. R. E. Stahl, A. Friedman-Kien, R. Dubin, M. Marmor, and S. Zolla-Pazner, Immunologic Abnormalities in Homosexual Men. Relationship to Kaposi's Sarcoma, Am J Med. 73:171 (1982).
4. E. O. Rasmussen, K. D. Cooper, K. Kang, C. R. White, D. H. Regan, and J. M. Hanifin, Immunosuppression in a Homosexual Man with Kaposi's Sarcoma, J Am Acad Dermatol. 6:870 (1982).
5. P. H. Tsang, K. Tangnavarad, S. Solomon, and J. G. Bekesi, Modulation of T- and B-Lymphocyte Functions by Isoprinosine in Homosexual Subjects with Prodomata and Patients with Acquired Immune Deficiency Syndrome (AIDS), J. Clin. Immunology. 4:469 (1984).
6. F. Lew, P. Tsang, S. Solomon, I. J. Selikoff, and J. G. Bekesi, Natural killer cell function and modulation by αIFN and IL2 in AIDS patients and prodromal subjects. J Clin Lab Immunol. 14:115 (1984).
7. S. E. Krown, F. X. Real, S. Cunningham-Rundles, P. Myskowski, B. Koziner, S. Fein, A. Mittelmen, H. F. Oettgen, and B. Safai, Preliminary observations on the effect of recombinant leukocyte A interferon in homosexual men with Kaposi's sarcoma, N. Engl J Med. 308:107 (1983).
8. A. H. Rook, H. Masur, H. C. Lane, W. Frederick, T. Kasanhara, A. M. Macher, J. Y. Djeu, J. F. Manischewitz, L. Jackson, A. S. Fauci and G. V. Quinnan, Interleukin-2 enhances the depressed natural killer and cytomegalovirus-specific cytotoxic activities of lymphocytes from patients with the Acquired Immune Deficiency Syndrome, J. Clin Invest. 72:398 (1983).
9. R. B. Herberman, Immunoregulation and natural killer cells, Mol Immunol. 19:1313 (1982).

10. H. C. Lane, H. Masur, L. C. Edgar, G. Whalen, A. H. Rook, and A. S. Fauci, Abnormalities of B-Cell Activation and Immunoregulation in Patients with the Acquired Immunodeficiency Syndrome, Engl. J Med. 309:453 (1983).
11. H. Ikram, A. M. Prince, and L. N. Baker, Cytomegalovirus (CMV) antibody in male homosexuals: A source for CMV immune globulin, Vox Sang, 44:173 (1983).
12. R. A. Coutinno, N. Lelie, P. Albrecht-Van-Lent, E. E. Reerink-Brongers, L. Stootjesdijk, P. Dees, J. Nivard, J. Huisman, and H. W. Reesink, Efficacy of a heat inactivated hepatitis B vaccine in male homosexuals: Outcome of a placebo controlled dougle blind trial, Br Med J. (Clin Res) 286:1305 (1983).
13. W. L. Drew, M. A. Conant, R. C. Miner, E. S. Huang, J. L. Ziegler, J. R. Groundwater, J. H. Gullett, P. Volberding, D. I. Abrams, and L. Mintz, Cytomegalovirus and Kaposi's sarcoma in young homosexual men, Lancet 2:125 (1982).
14. K. A. Fawaz, and D. S. Matloff, Viral hepatitis in homosexual men, Gastroenterology 81:537 (1981).
15. J. Sonnabend, S. S. Witkin, and D. T. Purtilo, Acquired Immunodeficiency Syndrome, Opportunistic Infections, and Malignancies in Male Homosexuals. A Hypothesis of Etiologic Factors in Pathogenesis, JAMA 249:2370 (1983).
16. M. Essex, M. F. McLane, T. H. Lee, L. Falk, C. W. S. Howe, J. I. Mullins, C. Cabradilla, and D. P. Francis, Antibodies to cell membrane antigesn associated with human T-cell leukemia virus in patients with AIDS, Science, 220:859 (1983).
17. E. P. Gelmann, M. Popovic, D. Blayney, H. Masw, G. Sighu, R. E. Stahl, and R. C. Gallo, Proviral DNA of a retrovirus, human T-cell leukemia virus, in two patients with AIDS. Science 220:862 (1983).
18. R. C. Gallo, P. S. Sarin, E. P. Gelmann, M. Robert-Guroff, E. Richardson, V. S. Kalyanaraman, D. Mann, G. D. Sighu, R. E. Stahl, S. Zolla-Pazner, J. Leibowitch, and M. Popovic, Isolation of human T-cell leukemia virus in Acquired Immune Deficiency Syndrome (AIDS), Science 220:865 (1983).
19. F. Barre-Sinoussi, J. C. Chermann, F. Rey, M. T. Nugeyre, S. Chamaret, J. Gruest, C. Dauguet, C. Anler-Blin, F. Vizinet-Brun, C. Rouzioux, W. Rozenbaum, and L. Montagnier, Isolation of a T-lymphotropic retrovirus from a patient at risk for Acquired Immune Deficiency Syndrome (AIDS), Science 220:868 (1983).
20. I. Montagnier, J. C. Chermann, and F. Barre-Sinoussi, A new human T-lymphotropic retrovirus: characterization and possible role in lymphadenopathy and Acquired Immune Deficiency Syndrome. Cold Spring Harbor: The Cancer Cell 3. (in press) (1985).
21. E. Vilmer, C. Rouzioux, A. Fischer, J. C. Chermann, F. Barre-Sinoussi, C. Gazengel, C. Dauguet, P. Manigne, and C. Griscelli, Isolation of New Lymphotropic Retrovirus from Two Siblings with Haemophilia B, One with AIDS. Lancet 3:753 (1984).
22. S. S. Witkin, and J. Sonnaben, Immune Responses to Spermatozoa in Homosexual Men. Fertil Steril 39:337 (1983).
23. T. Ginsberg, and A. J. Glasky, Inosiplex: An immuno-modulation model for the treatment of viral disease. Ann NY Acad Sci. 284: 128 (1977).
24. J. W. Hadden, C. Lopez, R. J. O'Reilly, and E. M. Hadden, Levamisole and inosiplex: Antiviral agents with immunopotentiating action. Ann NY Acad Sci 284:139 (1977).
25. J. M. Rojo, G, Ogida, and M. P. Portoles, Enhancement and restoration of contact sensitivity reactions by isoprinosine, J Immunopharmacol 5:231 (1982).

26. A. Portoles, G. Ojida, J. M. Rojo, M. P. Portoles, and I. Barasovin, Modulating effects of isoprinosine on lymphocyte proliferative response under immunodepression conditions. J Immunopharmacol 5: 245 (1983).
27. C. Balestrino, E. Montesorro, A. Nocera, M. Ferrarini, and T. Hoffman, Augmentation of human peripheral blood natural killer activity by methisoprinol. J Bio Resp Mod 2:577 (1983).
28. J. Wybran J. P. Famaey, R. Gortz, I. Dab, A. Malfroot, and T. Appelboom, Inosiplex (isoprinosine): A review of its immunological and clinical effects in disease. Adv Pharmacol Ther II 6:123 (1982).
29. K. Y. Tsang, H. H. Fudenberg, and G. M. P. Galbraith, In vitro augmentation of interleukin-2 production and lymphocytes with the Tac antigen marker in patients with AIDS. N Engl J Med 310:987 (1984).

INTERFERON AND INTERLEUKIN-2 THERAPY OF KAPOSI'S SARCOMA

P.A. Volberding, C.B. Wofsy and D.I. Abrams

San Francisco General Hospital, AIDS Clinic
995 Potrero Ave., San Francisco, CA 94110

INTRODUCTION

It is difficult to treat Kaposi's sarcoma by conventional therapies in the setting of immune deficiency such as the acquired immunodeficiency syndrome (AIDS), because this treatment may cause further immune suppression. In AIDS, cytotoxic chemotherapy may, for example, increase the risk of opportunistic infections such as Pneumocystis pneumonia. Thus, this therapy, even if successful against the tumor, may potentially shorten survival. Because of these factors, experimental therapy with immune modulating agents has been particularly attractive in AIDS-related Kaposi's sarcoma. The two agents receiving most attention have been recombinant alpha interferon and recombinant interleukin-2. These will be the subject of this review. The results will be preliminary because the disease itself is so new and because many of the clinical trials of these agents are still in progress.

KAPOSI'S SARCOMA - CLINICAL PERSPECTIVES

Kaposi's sarcoma itself is not a new disease. Prior to AIDS, the principal affected populations in the United States were elderly men of Jewish or Mediterranean descent or patients with exogenous immunosuppression especially following renal transplantation(1,2). While Kaposi's sarcoma in AIDS is histologically indistinguishable from other settings, its clinical course is unique. While Kaposi's sarcoma in the elderly usually remains confined to the skin of the lower extremities and follows a relatively indolent course, the same tumor in AIDS is characterized by widespread cutaneous and visceral dissemination, rapid progression and early mortality either as a direct result of the tumor or from opportunistic infections associated with the underlying immunodeficiency(3).

No generally useful staging system for AIDS-related KS has been developed, but reports suggest that those clinical features which suggest more advanced immune deterioration are associated with a poor prognosis in patients with Kaposi's sarcoma(4,5). Principal among these are the presence of associated lymphoma-like B symptoms (unexplained night sweats, fevers, and weight loss) as well as elevations of the erythrocyte sedimentation rate, neutropenia or severe anemia.

THERAPY OF KAPOSI'S SARCOMA PRIOR TO AIDS

Traditional Kaposi's sarcoma has been responsive to several chemotherapeutic agents, especially vinca alkaloids. Therapy for Kaposi's sarcoma in African populations prior to AIDS has also resulted in a dramatic response to many cytotoxic agents(6).

A group of patients with Kaposi's sarcoma prior to AIDS which is of great interest for the current epidemic are those patients with tumor following renal transplantation and exogenous immunosuppression. A variety of reports confirm the high rate of Kaposi's sarcoma following renal transplantation(7,8) and further demonstrate an often dramatic tumor regression following discontinuation of these immunosuppressive medications. For these reasons, it is widely believed that if therapies could be developed to restore the relative immune competence in patients with AIDS, that this would be sufficient to control further progression or cause actual tumor regression. Of drugs available with immune modulatory possibilities, two that have received the broadest clinical application are recombinant alpha interferon and recombinant interleukin-2.

CLINICAL TRIALS OF RECOMBINANT ALPHA-INTERFERON

Alpha-interferon is an attractive agent to apply to AIDS-associated Kaposi's sarcoma for several reasons. Among these are its antiviral actions, its immune modulating activity, and its antiproliferative capability(9). The antiviral actions of alpha-interferon, while incompletely studied with respect to the causative AIDS retrovirus, provide a rationale for applications in AIDS. Similarly, the immune stimulating and antiproliferative activities also provide a rationale for this drug for a rapidly progressing tumor such as Kaposi's sarcoma appearing in the setting of immune deficiencies.

Clinical trials with alpha-interferon in AIDS-related Kaposi's sarcoma have been undertaken by numerous investigators. While some trials have used non-recombinant drug, more recent studies have focused on recombinant human alpha-interferon.

Clinical trials of recombinant human alpha-interferon (Schering Corporation) were begun in collaboration with the University of California, San Francsico, and the University of California, Los Angeles, in 1982. In the first trial, 10 patients from each institution were randomized to receive either a low or high dose of this drug. The low dose arm consisted of one million units alpha-interferon per meter square body surface area. It was administered subcutaneously on 5 consecutive days on alternate weeks for a minimum of two months. In contrast, the patients receiving high-dose alpha-interferon in these trials received 50 million units per meter square body surface area intravenously on the same schedule. Patients who showed antitumor response were allowed to continue on a lower maintenance dose for prolonged periods of time.

The results of this experience with alpha interferon have been previously published(10) and demonstrate several important points. The first is that the drug is, at least in high doses, capable of inducing regression of AIDS-associated Kaposi's sarcoma. Four of 10 patients treated with the high-dose arm had an objective response compared with 2 in the low-dose therapy. While this response to with high-dose alph-interferon is encouraging and comparable to that seen with cytotoxic chemotherapy such as vinblastine, no clear immunologic improvement was detected, and the drug was associated with substantial, although tolerable, subjective toxicity. This toxicity consists primarily of a flu-like syndrome with fever, chills, headache, generalized weakness and anorexia. In all cases this resolved promptly following discontinuation of the drug and in many patients decreased in severity with continued drug use. Objective toxicity was not a major problem in this trial consisting primarily of transient neutropenia and elevations in serum transaminase levels.

Based on this experience, a larger trial was conducted involving approximately 30 patients from San Francisco General Hospital and 30 patients from the University of California, Los Angeles. In this study, all patients received 30 million units of recombinant alpha-interferon (Schering Corporation) subcutaneously 3 times every week. Again if response was seen, therapy was continued for longer periods.

Response to alpha-interferon in this and the previous study was evaluated by conventional oncologic criteria. Thus, a partial response consisted of a greater than 50% reduction in the number and size of cutaneous lesions. A complete disappearance of all lesions was considered a complete response. Some component of subjective assessment was also required to estimate the nodularity and pigmentation of index lesions.

In this trial, 64 patients were treated with subcutaneous alpha-interferon; their median age was 34 years, and all patients were homosexual or bisexual men. Approximately one-third had prior opportunistic infections, usually Pneumocystis pneumonia and one-half of all patients had prior B-symptoms. These are important as they are major factors predicting a more aggressive disease and a lower response to therapeutic intervention. Six patients had prior vinblastine chemotherapy and 2 patients had been previously treated with other forms of alpha-interferon.

The results of this trial were similar to those discussed previously. Of 64 patients, 3 complete responses were recorded and 16 partial responses. This response rate, about 30%, is again comparable to that seen with single-agent chemotherapy. When subsets of the enrolled patients without B-symptoms or previous opportunistic infections were studied, the overall response rate was higher, approximately 50%.

The toxicity of subcutaneous alpha-interferon in this trial was similar to that seen in our previous experience. Again, patients complained primarily of flu-like symptoms and again objective toxicity was limited and reversible.

The effect of prognostic variables on response rate was studied in some detail. When grouped by stage of tumor dissemination, those with more limited degrees of dissemination (Stages A and B) had a higher response rate than those with more advanced stages. These results are demonstrated in Table I. Also, when grouped by presence or absence of B-symptoms or previous opportunistic infection, differences were detected, Table II. For example, patients who were asymptomatic responded in 50% of cases while those patients with previous B-symptoms had an 18% response rate. This is significant with a P value of less than .05. While not significant, a similar difference was detected for the effect of previous opportunistic infections. Here, patients without previous opportunistic infection had a response rate of 37% compared with a response rate of 19% in those with prior opportunistic infections.

TABLE I

RESPONSE TO IFN BY STAGE

STAGE		RESPONDERS/TOTAL
A	INDOLENT CUTANEOUS	11/28 (39%)
B	INDOLENT VISCERAL	8/19 (42%)
C	AGGRESSIVE CUTANEOUS	1/11 (9%)
D	AGGRESSIVE VISCERAL	0/3 (0%)
	A + B VS. C + D $p < 0.05$	
	A + C VS. B + D $p = 0.85$	

TABLE II

RESPONSE TO IFN BY SYMPTOMS OR PRIOR OI

CATEGORY		RESPONSE/TOTAL
A	ASYMPTOMATIC	15/32 (50%)
B	FEVER AND/OR WEIGHT LOSS	5/29 (18%) $p < .05$
-	WITHOUT OI	17/45 (37%)
+	WITH OI	3/16 (19%) p = NS

In addition to antitumor response, a major index of activity for any immunologically active drug in AIDS is the incidence of opportunsitic infections following drug therapy. In our trial, as has been true in other reports, responders are clearly different than nonresponders. While opportunistic infections were seen in 5 nonresponders to alpha-interferon, infections were seen in only one patient with an objective antitumor response. Following interferon therapy, this trend continued with 11 opportunistic infections in nonresponders and only 2 in those responding to the drug.

While conclusions regarding the role of alpha-interferon in AIDS-related Kaposi's sarcoma must still be somewhat guarded, we feel that we have demonstrated that this drug has activity and can induce objective responses. Overall, approximately 30 to 40% of patients achieved an objective response, but this rate could be increased by more careful patient selection, especially limiting these trials to those patients without previous B-symptoms or previous opportunistic infections. In this way, an objective response rate of approximately 50 to 60% is probably achievable. While these response rates are encouraging, subjective toxicities in these trials have limited maximum doses. In the future, it will be desirable to confirm our findings in other centers and as much more is currently known concerning the role of retroviruses in causing immune deficiency, it will be important to include monitoring for antiviral activity against these viruses with clinical trials.

RECOMBINANT INTERLEUKIN-2

As was the case with trials of recombinant alpha-interferon, interleukin-2 provides several rationales for clinical trials in AIDS-associated Kaposi's sarcoma. Interleukin-2 is a necessary growth factor for T-lymphocytes and interleukin-2 production is deficient in lymphocytes isolated from patients with AIDS(11). Even more strikingly, when lymphocytes are purified from AIDS patients, incubation with interleukin-2 restores functional activities such as mitogenic responsiveness to normal or near-normal levels(12). For these reasons, clinical trials of recombinant interleukin-2 in patients with AIDS were initiated. Again the hope was that this drug would be effective in restoring some degree of immune competence which would then indirectly result in antineoplastic action.

Since the initiation of our clinical trials, a major potential problem has arisen. It is now apparent that interleukin-2 is a potent stimulator, not only of normal T-lymphocytes, but potentially also that sub-fraction infected with the AIDS-associated retrovirus. Because retroviral expression is increased during cellular division, administration of interleukin-2 may accelerate _in vivo_ viral production resulting in a more rapid recruitment of previously uninfected cells. This possibility is serious as adverse immunological consequences could result.

The goals of our clinical trials of recombinant interleukin-2 (Cetus Corporation) were to conduct a dose-finding trial monitoring toxicity as well as immunologic responsiveness. In our trial, patients are divided into two groups, A and B. Those in group A have only Kaposis's sarcoma while those in group B have a history of recovery from an AIDS-associated opportunistic infection in the presence or absence of Kaposi's sarcoma. Dose escalation of groups of patients in group A and B are planned with doses ranging from very low to expected maximum tolerable dose. No intrapatient dose escalations are planned and all patients are treated with intravenous infusions of recombinant interleukin-2 three times weekly for eight weeks. At the end of 8 weeks, patients are assessed. If antineoplastic activity is observed, maintenance therapy is allowed, otherwise patients are removed from therapy at 8 weeks and monitored subsequently for survival, rate of opportunistic infection, and immunologic characterizations.

At this point our results are extremely preliminary with only approximately 50% of expected patients on trial. With the doses used to date, 1000 and 10,000 units/m^2 body surface area, no objective Kaposi's sarcoma responses have been recorded. While patients have developed Pneumocystis pneumonia while on study, in most cases these patients had a previous history of opportunistic infections. At this point, there has been no evidence of adverse immunologic or clinical effects and toxicity has been minimal. There has been at the same time then a real but minor improvement in in vitro immunologic testing of study patients. Of these tests, PHA responsivenes appears to be more sensitive to interleukin-2 with no clear trends yet seen with clinical response or response by dose.

CONCLUSIONS AND FUTURE DIRECTIONS

A great deal has been learned in the past 3 years about the immunological status and immune therapy of patients with AIDS-associated Kaposi's sarcoma. Our own trials and those others indicate a role for recombinant alpha-interferon with objective response rates approaching those of several chemotherapeutic agents. Results with interleukin-2 are, at this point, extremely preliminary and no conclusions should be drawn. We would anticipate that in the future major efforts will be directed at developing drugs effective against the causative agent of AIDS. As antiviral therapies are explored, their role in different patient subsets will need to be tested. While antiviral therapy alone may, for example, be adequate for patients prior to the development of the severe immunologic deterioration, further adjuvant therapies may be necessary if this severe immune deterioration has occurred. In this latter group of patients, antiviral therapy without simultaneous therapy to restore immune competence may be inadequate. For these reasons, combinations of antiviral drugs with drugs such as recombinant interleukin-2 may be envisioned. Similarly, the role of recombinant alpha-interferon is likely to change. As more is learned of its antiviral capabilities, trials using a variety of doses and schedules to optimize this action may be interesting.

While successful therapy of AIDS remains an elusive goal, optimism is possible because of the rapid increase in our understanding of this disease. Hopefully with continued clinical research following basic in vitro observation and testing, agents will be found capable of a significant impact in this otherwise almost uniformly fatal disease.

REFERENCES

1. B. Safai, R. A. Good, Kaposi's sarcoma: A review in recent developments. Clin Bulletin 10:62-69 (1980).
2. P. H. O'Brien and R. D. Brasfield, Kaposi's sarcoma. Cancer 19:1497-1502 (1966).
3. K. B. Hymes, T. Cheung, J. B. Green, et al, Kaposi's sarcoma in homosexual men. Report of 8 cases, Lancet ii:598-600 (Sept. 1981).
4. R. Kriegel, L. Laubenstein, F. Muggia, Kaposi's sarcoma: A new staging classification. Cancer Treatment Reports 67:531-534 (1983).
5. P. Volberding, K. Kaslo, M. Bilk, et al, Prognostic factors in staging Kaposi's sarcoma in the acquired immunodeficiency syndrome. Proceedings American Society of Clinical Oncology, p 19, (1984).
6. P. Volberding, M. A. Conant, R. B. Stricker, B. J. Lewis, Chemotherapy in advanced Kaposi's sarcoma: Implications for current cases in homosexual men. Am J Med 74:652-656 (1983).
7. J. H. Siegel, R. Janis, J. Alper, et al, Disseminated Kaposi's sarcoma - appearance after human renal aligraft operation. JAMA 207:1493-1496 (1969).
8. B. D. Myers, E. Kessler, J. Levi, et al, Kaposi's sarcoma in kidney transplant patients. Arch Int Med 133:307-311 (1974).
9. S. E. Krown, F. X. Real, S. Cunningham-Rundles, et al, Preliminary observations on the effect of recombinant leukocyte interferon in homosexual men with Kaposi's sarcoma. New Engl J Med 308:1071-1076 (1983).
10. J. E. Groopman, M. S. Gottlieb, J. Goodman, et al, Recombinant alpha-2 interferon therapy of Kaposi's sarcoma associated with acquired immunodeficiency syndrome. Ann Int Med 100:671-677 (1984).
11. K. Welte, N. Ciobanun, G. Kruger, et al, Impaired interleukin-2 production in response to PHA and OKT3 antibody in male homosexuals with acquired immunodeficiency syndrome: in vitro restoration of T-cell proliferation by highly purified interleukin-2, in: "AIDS, The Epidemic of Kaposi's Sarcoma and Opportunistic Infections," A. E. Friedman-Kien, L. J. Laubenstein, eds., Masson Publishing U.S.A. Inc., New York, 199-205, (1983).
12. A. H. Rook, H. Masur, H. C. Lane, et al, Interleukin-2 enhances the depressed natural killer in cytomegalovirus specific cytotoxic activities of lymphocytes from patients with the acquired immunodeficiency syndrome. J Clin Invest 72:398-403 (1983).

CYTOTOXIC CHEMOTHERAPY IN KAPOSI'S SARCOMA

Steven A. Armentrout

University of California, Irvine
Irvine, CA 92717

Kaposi's sarcoma, recognized in the Western Hemisphere as an indolent malignant cutaneous disease affecting primarily elderly males of Jewish extraction, has in recent years been the principle malignancy associated with acquired immune deficiency syndrome (AIDS). The wide-spread cutaneous lesions are frequently associated with viseral involvement, particularly in the pulmonary and gastrointestinal systems. The early cutaneous manifestations of Kaposi's sarcoma appear to respond to the administration of interferon. This biologic has not, however, afforded permanent control in this disease. A variety of chemotherapeutic regimens have been employed in an effort to control advanced cutaneous and viseral Kaposi's sarcoma (1-7). The use of cytotoxic chemotherapy has resulted in a substantial percentage of partial and complete responses in the malignant lesions. The duration of both complete and partial responses has, however, proved disappointingly short. Another theoretical as well as practical disadvantage of cytotoxic chemotherapy, has been a further suppression of the immune system in the patient with AIDS. Although frequently difficult to quantitate, this appears to have resulted in a further increase in systemic life threatening infections by both common and opportunistic pathogens. Recent trials of chemotherapy employing both cytotoxic chemotherapy and biologic response modifiers, although too early to evaluate, seem to produce results similar to cytotoxic chemotherapy alone.

Two commonly employed chemotherapeutic regimens are VP 16-213 administered on three successive days monthly, and a combination chemotherapy including adriamycin, bleomycin and vinblastine (ABV) administered in a 21 day cycle. Both of these cytotoxic regimens have produced significant numbers of partial and complete remissions but the duration of remissions have proved disappointingly short and the infectious complications limiting. The current study reports the results of nine patients with advanced Kaposi's sarcoma treated with an alternating program of VP 16-213 and AVB. This protocol was employed in an attempt to reduce toxicity and prolong remission duration.

The patients treated in the present series are male with an age range between 24 and 46. The median age was 31. All the patients were sexually active homosexuals and had prior or concurrent laboratory documentation of the abnomalities associated with the aquired immune deficiency syndrome. All patients had a history of frequent infection, seven with opportunistic pathogens and three with pneumocystis carinii pneumonia. Four of the nine

Table 1. Chemotherapy

42 Day Cycle		
Day 1,3,5	VP 16-213	150 mg/m^2
Day 22	Adriamycin	30 mg/m^2
	Bleomycin	30 u
	Vinblastine	5 mg/m^2

Dosage modification - 25% reduction in cytotoxic drug dosage if nadir granulocyte count 1200.

patients had extensive cutaneous lesions without documented viseral involvement. Five patients had documented viseral involvement in addition to cutaneous disease. One patient had pulmonary lesions and four had gastrointestinal lesions at the time of presentation. Two patients with gastrointestinal lesions had a history of severe recurrent gastrointestinal bleeding with symptomatic anemia which required periodic transfusion. All patients had disease staging which included physical examination, radiographic and enteroscopic gastrointestinal examination, chest x-ray and/or computerized tomography of the chest, complete blood counts and bone marrow examination when indicated, and serum chemistries including hepatic and renal function tests. All areas of documented disease or documented laboratory abnormalities were examined routinely. Other radiographic and endoscopic examinations were performed where indicated by symptoms or abnormal physical findings.

Chemotherapy was administered on a 42 day schedule with VP 16-213, 150 mg/m^2 administered on days 1, 3, and 5, and adriamycin 30 mg/m^2, bleomycin 30 u, and vinblastine 5 mg/m^2 administered on day 22. Weekly blood counts were obtained to determine nadir counts of granulocytes and platelets. Dosage modification of 25% in either VP 16-213 or adriamycin and vinblastine was instituted if the nadir granulocyte count was less than 1,200 mm^3. The chemotherapy protocol is outlined in Table 1.

A complete response was defined as a complete disappearance of all evidence of Kaposi's sarcoma in all involved sites. A partial response was defined as greater than 50 and less than 100 percent resolution of the lesions in all areas of involvement. Stable disease was defined as less than 50 percent resolution of all lesions lasting greater than one cycle (42 days) or a mixed response in which the mean of regression was greater than 0 and less than 50 percent during this time period. Progressive disease was defined as a greater than 25 percent increase in measurable lesions in a one month period.

No complete remissions were observed in the nine patients currently entered in this study. Three patients demonstrated a partial remission. All of these patients are currently alive at 5, 11, and 13 months from the initiation of cytotoxic chemotherapy. All remain currently in partial remission and in one patient, the lesions continue to regress at five months. Five patients have demonstrated stable disease or a mixed response. Two of the patients are alive at 3 and 11 months respectively. Three patients died of associated infectious complications at 5, 7, and 9 months respectively. All these patients remained with either stable disease or a continued mixed response. One patient demonstrated progressive disease while on cytotoxic chemotherapy. He died three months following

Table 2. Response

Complete Response	0/9	
Partial Response	3/9	3 alive (5,11,13 mo)
Stable Disease	5/9	2 alive (3,11 mo) 3 dead (5,7,9 mo)
No Response	1/9	1 dead (3 mo)

the initiation of chemotherapy with complications associated with Kaposi's sarcoma. Two patients with stable disease or a mixed response had episodes of gastrointestinal hemorrhage requiring transfusion during the period of demonstrated disease stability. One of these patients died subsequently of infectious complications, the other patient is still alive requiring episodic transfusions for gastrointestinal hemorrhage. The results of this chemotherapy are summarized in Table 2.

This chemotherapeutic program was well tolerated by all nine patients. The principal direct drug related toxicity was due to bone marrow suppression. All nine patients showed some degree of leukopenia. This leukopenia was mild to moderate and no patient demonstrated a total granulocyte count at nadir below 1,000 mm^2. No patients demonstrated life threatening leukopenia at any time during the course of their therapy. Three of the nine patients demonstrated a mild to moderate depression in platelet count. At nadir, no thrombocyte count was below 80,000 mm^2 and no episodes of bleeding were attributed either to thrombocytopenia or thrombocytopathia. Mild anemia was seen in two of the nine patients and in one patient, severe symptomatic anemia appeared on three occasions. The patient demonstrating symptomatic anemia had repeated gastrointestinal hemorrhages both prior to and during therapy. This patient was transfused frequently and at no time had platelet depression which was felt to be contributory. Gastrointestinal symptoms were observed in four of the nine patients and included anorexia, nausea and an occasional episode of vomiting in the immediate post-therapy period. None of these patients required anti-emetic therapy except in the 24 hours immediately following the administration of ABV. There was no evidence of pulmonary toxicity manifested either by symptoms, x-ray changes, or blood gas determinations in any of the patients. One patient had a history of recurrent severe pulmonary infections. This patient who had demonstrated stable disease had a decrease in pulmonary function and deteriorating pulmonary symptomatology attributed to advancing infection with atypical myco-bacteria during the final month of life. The toxicity of this chemotherapeutic program is summarized in Table 3.

In this small series of patients with advanced Kaposi's sarcoma, cytotoxic chemotherapy produced either partial remission or stable disease in the majority of individuals. The median duration of response or in stable disease was greater than eight months. In this series, the median duration of survival was greater than nine months. Of the five patients remaining alive all continue to demonstrate stability of their Kaposi's sarcoma. In only one of the four patients who expired, was death attributed to complications of Kaposi's sarcoma. Despite these encouraging preliminary results, considerable morbidity and mortality resulted from intercurrent infection. It was difficult to determine whether these patients demonstrated

Table 3. Toxicity

	Grade 0 - 2	Grade 3 - 4
Leukopenia	9/9	0/9
Thrombocytopenia	3/9	0/9
Anemia	2/9	1/9*
Pulmonary	0/9	0/9
Gastrointestinal	4/9	0/9
Other	-	-

*Repeated gastrointestinal hemmorhage.

an increase in number and severity of infections following the administration of cytotoxic therapy, but these proved the most significant complicating factor in managing all nine. While the use of aggressive cytotoxic chemotherapy seems to provide short term benefit for patients with advanced Kaposi's sarcoma, it is quite evident that in the absence of therapy directed toward modification of the basic immune deficiency, encouraging long-term results will be difficult to obtain. Further investigations will be necessary to demonstrate whether this approach employing alternating cytotoxic chemotherapeutic programs coupled with biologic response modifiers will be superior to less aggressive approaches in the management of advanced Kaposi's sarcoma.

1. B. Safai, Clinical features of Kaposi's sarcoma/aquired immune deficiency syndrome and its management, Antibiot-Chemother. 32:54-70 (1983).
2. A. C. Bayley, Aggressive Kaposi's sarcoma in Zambia, 1983, Lancet 1:1318-20 (1984).
3. A. Poulsen, B. Hultberg, K. Thomsen, and G. L. Wantzin, Regression of Kaposi's sarcoma in AIDS after treatment with dapsone, Lancet 1:560 (1984).
4. K. H. Antman, L. Nadler, E. J. Mark, D. L. Montella, P. Kirkpatrick, and J. Halpern, Primary Kaposi's sarcoma of the lung in an immunocompetent 32-year-old heterosexual white man, Cancer 54: 1696-8 (1984).
5. M. Markowitz, C. Metroka, and A. Moore, VP 16-213 (Etoposide) and bleomycin in the treatment of Kaposi's sarcoma, Proc Annu Meet Am Soc Clin Oncol 3:58 (1984).
6. K. K. Ketiku and F. A. Durosinmi-Etti, The treatment of Kaposi's sarcoma by combination chemotherapy in Nigeria, Clin Radiol 35:155-8 (1984).
7. B. Lewis, D. Abrams, J. Ziegler, M. Conant, G. Gee, I. Silverberg, and P. Volberding, Single agent or combination chemotherapy of Kaposi's sarcoma (KS) in aquired immune deficiency syndrome (AIDS), Proc Am Soc Clin Oncol 2:C-232 (1983).

CONFERENCE SUMMATION

Robert A. Good

Oklahoma Medical Research Foundation

Oklahoma City, Oklahoma

This meeting has been an extraordinary experience and I believe all participants in the International Conference on AIDS Associated Syndromes feel deeply indebted to the many speakers for the clarity of their presentations and the fine slides and data they have shown us. Particularly, we must appreciate Dr. Sudhir Gupta's effort in organizing the conference. We appreciate as well support by the Newport Pharmaceutical Company that made holding this important meeting at such a crucial time possible. Particularly, we must thank Dr. Alvin Glasky, President of Newport Pharmaceuticals, for his enthusiastic support both for this conference and his active participation in the rapidly developing field of immunopharmacology.

When I first heard there was going to be another conference on AIDS to comprise a day and a half, my reaction was--"not another conference on AIDS." But as the conference developed, the subject turned out to be very special. We have dealt primarily with the AIDS Related Complex (ARC). Much new information has been presented and I feel personally enriched by what has come forth here. We launched the symposium with a series of papers that showed very clearly what ARC is like, clinically. The manifestations of ARC were described and the manifestations elucidated. The patients usually have lymphadenopathy, weight loss, night sweats, fever, and a variety of immunological defects. The presentations established once and for all that the ARC although often quite stable, can progress directly into frank AIDS. This was shown in the presentations of by Gottlieb and Pinching, Abrams and others. Once AIDS has developed from this complex, the AIDS syndrome that develops behaves just like all forms of AIDS that develop as a primary disease and has a very high morbidity and virtually a uniform lethality. This information, which is both important and new, is also most threatening. This fact needed to be established and now has been ascertained beyond doubt.

The initial presentations and some presentations that followed showed that there may be little red warning flags of what is to come for the individual patient. None of the warning signs are definitive. Although they may indicate the likelihood of ultimate progression to AIDS, none of the warning signs or laboratory findings, not even elevated levels of acid-labile alpha-interferon uniformly signals that progression of ARC to AIDS will occur. Many of the patients with ARC seem to remain stable for prolonged periods even though they have significant and measurable immunodeficiencies. Further, it seems implied from the evidence presented, that AIDS plus ARC together represent only the tip of an iceberg. Many patients are infected with the causative virus and most of these do not even express clinical disease. Thus, subclinical infection exists, and thus too immunity must occur, although I have not seen unequivocal evidence of the latter. The full range of possibilities appears to be like those seen with many other virus infections and range from subclinical to regressor disease to ARC to AIDS. We don't yet know nor can we ascertain what will happen to any person who has been infected with the virus. This is especially true for viral influences over a long period. Because the virus in present form is so new time has not yet been sufficient to clarify these issues. Live animals and humans often have great difficulty getting rid of viruses--it seems possible that we will see other consequences of infection with this retrovirus that will cause unforeseen troubles in the future. Nonetheless, I think it likely, in thinking of potential therapies and of the possibilities of immunization, that most infected people handle infection with the AIDS virus very well and do not express frank ARC or AIDS. Those infected infrequently may forthwith develop AIDS. Alternatively they may develop a stable ARC. They may develop ARC that progresses to AIDS. They may even get ARC and gradually get well. Or they may be infected without developing evidence of disease. Whether they develop a firm immunity has not yet been established but seems a likely possibility.

I think we have learned from this meeting not only the threatening information that ARC can progress to AIDS itself, but of manifestations that predict this awful sequence. Very low levels of the T_4 helper lymphocyte population, very low T_4/T_8 ratios, marked lymphopenia, are ominous signs. But none are definitive. Knowing the virus etiology of AIDS and ARC and the range of clinical expression thus far defined makes me feel certain that immunization against AIDS can be worked out. Important to this conference is evidence that serological analysis can serve as with other virus infections to recognize patients who are infected and those who have been infected and virological study reveals quite definitively those who are infected but it is not an exclusive parameter. It was nice to begin to see new certainties appear now that serological analyses and virus isolation are a regular part of a proper analyses of patients. These virological and serological contributions reflect the crucial efforts of the French scientists led by Duc Montonier from the Pasteur Institute, who first isolated the virus so rapidly, and the tremendous reinforcement afforded by the Americans led by Robert Gallo. I, for one, am convinced that the LAV-HTLV-III virus or viruses represent the true cause of AIDS and also the cause of ARC. No alternative to explain current findings need be sought in my view. The virus may not be the only underlying influence on the immunologic system of these patients, but it is the causative agent, and without it we wouldn't have AIDS--it is the sole etiologic determinant of the disease ultimately expressed as AIDS or ARC. Complications on the other hand may involve other viruses, combinations of other viruses just as they may involve bacterias, fungi and protozoa. But the root cause is now known and it is the LAV-HTLV-III agent.

As with so many diseases, everyone who studies AIDS looks at the elephant a bit differently but now we all must try to relate our perspective of pathogenesis to the root cause in the LAV or HTLV-III virus infection. The papers on ARC, its natural history, progression to AIDS, and the association with other infections all fit the perspective of this disease as a viral disease. It is the AIDS virus, LAV or HTLV-III that has a tropism for the T_4 subpopulation of lymphocytes. It infects and destroys these cells producing overt infection with immunodeficiency ARC and even subclinical infection. This virus infection is an awful one but knowing the cause should hurry along the solution to this life-threatening problem. It is the biggest step which could have been taken. Risk factors and determinants of progression as presented by several essayists, and even figures reflecting the frequency of progression over time will be helpful in the future, and all were presented here.

It may be possible to sharpen even further and finally to have simple means of assessing progress of our patients from ARC to AIDS or from ARC to good health. With such life threatening consequences of this evaluation it is important that we sharpen our ability to predict if we cannot at the moment do much to control progression. Further, sharpening is just that. From what was presented, it may no longer be essential to do repeatedly the extensive immunoparameter studies to evaluate ARC in order to predict progress to AIDS or to good health. Dr. Hershey, Dr. Krown, when she was considering Kaposi's sarcoma, and Dr. S. Cunningham-Rundles all presented information on the appearance of cytotoxic effectors which suggest that the apparent loss or absence of such effectors can be helpful in predicting the direction the infection will take or is taking.

Is there anything that can be done about AIDS, ARC and the progression of ARC to AIDS right now? Did this conference bring forward any hopeful information to suggest directions that may be developed to stop progression of the infection to AIDS or the lethal progression once AIDS has appeared? I was impressed from several of the clinical trials reported that in a certain proportion of the patients' treatment with immunomodulators, eg interferon, may have facilitated regression of the Kaposi's sarcoma in some patients. Unfortunately, the proportion of patients so helped was not commanding. Thirty-eight percent in the series of Susan Krown got better. Seventeen percent in another series had complete regressions and 15% in still another. Further, the responses observed with Kaposi's sarcoma were sometimes but not regularly major responses and they were occasionally accompanied by improvement in immunological functions. We still have no cure of the AIDS syndrome, but using only one of many possible interferons it looks like we may have made a small beginning in treating one of the several malignant complications, namely Kaposi's sarcoma. More encouraging was that the few successes were sometimes associated with improvement in the depressed, delayed allergic responses and in the proportion and number of T_4 cells or the T_4/T_8 ratios. Even the NK cell numbers and activity seemed to be improved by treatment in some patients. This beginning should form one cornerstone of foundation on which much more can be built. When you consider the findings reported together with evidence that when interferon therapy was used as a supplement to cytotoxic chemotherapeutic treatment encouraging results may be seen. Indeed, Susan Krown told us of her experience combining vincristine plus interferon, 11 of 18 Kaposi's patients showed major, albeit short-lived, remissions. Further, an additional 7 of 18 patients showed minor remissions. Thus, all or nearly all patients showed some response to this combination. This has to be taken as a good start. Dr. Armentrout, who has used cytotoxic chemotherapeutic agents extensively and has in the past used them with some value to treat classical Kaposi's sarcoma, showed that in the aggressive Kaposi's sarcoma associated with AIDS approximately 30% of the patients could be improved. None of these series is speaking of a true and reproducible cure. But it is important to remember that when Hodgkins disease, which we treat so effectively with combination treatment today, was treated with single chemotherapeutic agents the results revealed only temporary regressions. Later on combinations of chemotherapeutics plus irradiation and chemotherapeutic combinations like MOPP ultimately did result in cures. Perhaps combinations of immunofacilitators, immunomodulators, pro-host effectors together, or perhaps following other chemotherapeutic approaches that are directly injurious to the Kaposi's sarcoma tumor cells in these patients will be dramatically more helpful. I think it likely that single agents will never work well for AIDS but also contend that strategies or combinations of treatments may ultimately be developed that can work to cure this disease. The influences of interferon plus IL-2, plus certain thymic factors plus Newport's isoprinosine may be much better when used together than when any of these are used alone.

I thought Bekesi's contribution was especially notable. He used the completely non-toxic agent, isoprinosine, originally developed as an antiviral agent. He was able, with treatment lasting only one month, to produce dramatic influences on objective immunoparameters in patients with the AIDS Related Complex which were measurable and even showed progressive improvement over nearly one year. He observed significant beneficial effects on NK cell function, on the numbers and functions of cells of the T-helper population T_4, and on total lymphocyte numbers +11. All these improvements appeared to lead to continuing improvement of immunoparamenters over several months. The influences on several depressed lymphoid and immunologic parameters which of course must be confirmed with larger numbers of patients in multiple locations suggest that isoprinosine, a very safe drug, or other closely related agents may be developed into another cornerstone of a strategy for treating the AIDS Related Complex. This approach using a form of immunomodulation needs much more study. It also needs more critical evaluation and perhaps ultimate use, not only in AIDS and ARC but in other immunodepressing virus infections of man. I expect this toddling step will also look much better when it is coupled to other immunomodulatory treatments melded into imaginative strategies.

We should always look for surprises. One surprise was the strange association that Allen Goldstein told us about between ARC, AIDS and the putative thymic hormone Thymosine α_1 levels in the blood. Thymosin α_1 is a purified, genetically sequenced molecule which has been produced by biosynthetic techniques using recombinant DNA technology. It is thus a molecule which has been completely defined. From immunologic analysis it seemed at first as though thymosin α_1 levels were very high in AIDS. Such a finding would be confusing especially since the thymus is so completely involuted in these patients and levels of FTS or Thymulin have been shown by Incefy et al to be so low. But this thymosin α_1 reactive material is very high in concentration in blood of a few patients with AIDS but is regularly elevated in ARC. The elevations of these levels were also found in male homosexuals and in patients with AIDS itself but were less dramatic than the elevations in ARC. As it turns out, the active material does not appear to be true thymosine α_1 but rather a substance cross-reactive immunologically with thymosin α_1. Thus, in the serum of these patients, a molecule, immunologically similar but not identical to one of the thymus hormones, thymosin α_1 is present. His finding reminded me of observations that Bijan Safai made in my laboratories several years ago when we were studying his Mycosis fungoides patients with Dr. G. Incefy and Dr. J. Twomey. In the blood of patients with mycosis fungoides activity, that seemed to be a thymic hormone, was found to be present in very large amounts. Paradoxically, however, this material was present in especially high concentrations in octagenarians and even nonogenarians who have no demonstrable thymus or thymic hormones ordinarily. The factor present in blood seemed to be indistinguishable initially from FTS which French scientists, led by Bach and Dardenne had described. It didn't make much sense for very old people to have this thymic hormone in high levels. Indeed, thymulin is ordinarily unmeasurable after the age of 35-40 years. The factor present in such large amounts, while related to thymulin and thymopoietic turned out to be different from either and may be produced by the skin and related to but distinct from the putative thymic hormone. Actually it may be a product of the skin. Just what this factor is that has thymic hormone reactivity in patients with AIDS must be further studied because it does not fit and would be a most important determinant.

We must understand in chemical terms what produces the apparently incongruous data concerning thymosinα_1 and other thymic hormones in AIDS. All physical and morphological studies, and other hormone studies indicate that the thymus is destroyed dramatically or accidentally involuted early in the course of AIDS. What then is the chemistry and source of the cross-reactive material. These findings may ultimately help us to understand how thymosinα_1 may be helpful rather than harmful in patients with ARC. Arthur Gottlieb's findings may also be providing an indication that perhaps other thymic factors may be of benefit to patients with ARC or AIDS.

Since today's session is so fresh in our minds, and since the hour is getting late, I will not review details of this day's deliberations except to say that Dr. Markham and Dr. Burch in comprehensive and informative presentations have taught us new lessons about the association HTLV-III virus of Gallo and the lymphadenopathy associated virus of Luc Montonier. These viruses are closely related to one another but each is much, much more distantly related to other HTLV retroviruses of man. The latter of course have only recently and for the first time been associated with human malignancies. One must credit Hinuma et al from Kyoto and Gallo et al with demonstrating that these human retroviruses are associated with and the probable causes of leukemia in Western Kyushu in Japan and with leukemias or lymphomas in the Caribbean. The diseases caused by these first of the human retroviruses have thus far all been adult T-Cell lymphomas or leukemias. The AIDS agent is quite a different virus from each of these and thus represents a third human retrovirus which can cause disease. More recently we have heard that non-A non-B virus may also be a retrovirus. Thus, we are already well into the human retrovirus era and malignancies as well as immunodeficiencies and other origin diseases may all be the consequences just as with retroviruses of animals. Coming out of this conference and now pervading all of human cancer are findings which indicated that immunosurveillance against certain forms of cancer is not quite as moribund as Nossal has said but seems to me quite well resuscitated instead. Cancers and malignancies are very much a part of AIDS. The cancers that occur so frequently are Kaposi's sarcoma, B-Cell lymphomas, leukemias, squamous cell carcinomas of skin, mouth and tissues of cloacagenic origin as well as malignant melanomas. This is almost exactly the same group of cancers which have represented such major clinical threat in patients chemically immunosuppressed for organ transplantation. Cyclosporin has been especially prone to open the door to such cancers in humans. Patients who are born with primary immunodeficiencies also have too much cancer. We do not yet have the capacity to shut off the immunodeficiency of AIDS and so do not know how to prevent or treat the cancers effectively in these patients. By contrast in immunosuppressed patients Starzl has shown that simply stopping the suppression of immunity, eg in the cyclosporin-treated patients, is sufficient to induce them to completely reject their tumors.

Certainly also related to these findings is the increased frequency of occurrence of a related set of cancers in patients with certain primary immunodeficiency diseases of genetic origin. An increased frequency of tumors of B-cell origin and epithelial tumors of head and neck, GI tract and skin occur in these patients. In three situations immunorestoration appears to exert a telling influence on the cancers. When patients with Wiskott-Aldrich syndrome or Severe Combined Immunodeficiency, for example, have been cured of their immunodeficiency disease by marrow transplantation. Malignancies do not appear with such frequency as in patients who have not been effectively treated. Similarly, cessation of immunosuppression causes Kaposi's sarcoma to go away completely in transplanted patients after such manipulation and all of the other malignancies which develop in immunosuppressed patients regress when the immunosuppressive treatment is stopped.

These findings represent clinching evidence that immunosurveillance is for real and that under proper conditions the immunity systems can eliminate trillions of cancer cells, not just a few thousand cancer cells. All you have to do to get rid of these kinds of cancers is to stop suppressing the immunity system.

I was so impressed by the paper of Starzl and colleagues in Lancet last summer that I travelled to Pittsburgh and, with the pathologists who collaborated in this study, reviewed the regressions of the nearly 16 cancers in question. When Starzl and his associates quit suppressing the immunity system, B-Cell Lymphomas, Kaposi's sarcoma and even one case of Hodgkins disease melted away under the host immune assault. That was a very dramatic thing to see. There is no question in my mind that these tumors represent true cancers. Where properly studied, the tumors in immunosuppressed patients have been shown to be monoclonal expansions as shown first by Cleary. They are usually monoclonal expansions of the B lymphocytes, and are often attributable to influences of the EB virus. However, Kaposi's sarcoma which is related to CMV virus infection is also rejected in immunosuppressed patients if immunosuppressive treatment is stopped. Thus, there is little doubt that if we could inhibit the immunosuppression in patients with AIDS efficiently and effectively restore immunologic function, their regularly lethal cancers would either not develop or if developed would be rejected. It is a synergistic action of the HTLV-III-LAV plus the cytomegalovirus (CMV) combination that produces Kaposi's sarcoma in the AIDS patient and HTLV-III induced immunosuppression plus EBV infection produce B-Cell lymphomas in these patients. With the furious pace of studies generated from this focus of excitation we can be sure next time we have a symposium like this we will know much more about the intimate details of viral cause of cancer, the role of immunosuppression and how EBV and CMV viruses contribute to producing cancers in the immunosuppressed patients. I have stated earlier that I question whether Kaposi's sarcoma is a true malignancy. This tumor, that is certainly associated with the CMV, is surely a proliferative disease which almost certainly involves endothelial cells. It is also highly aggressive in these patients and may be lethal. Purtilo, with his extraordinary studies of patients with a lacunar immunodeficiency, has shown that the EBV DNA virus produces many malignancies and also produces other secondary immunodeficiencies in patients unable to marshall an effective cellular immune response against that virus. He has reviewed many of these manifestations here and has elucidated for us the contributions of the EB virus, in the pathogenesis of both B-Cell lymphomas and immunodeficiency. Dr. Greenspan also showed today how the EB virus plus papilloma virus may work together to produce the well-established, precancerous lesion called oral leukoplakia. Nonetheless, the apparently highly malignant and aggressive Kaposi's sarcoma which occurs in AIDS patients does not behave in nude mice, for example, like other true cancers and more evidence of its clonal nature is needed.

We also learned today that AIDS first appeared not in the homosexuals of America as everyone has thought but rather in Central Equitorial Africa. A thread of this origin already appeared in earlier discussions, but now I think we have even more convincing serological evidence that this is the case. We are left, as Dr. Markham pointed out, with the question of how the LAV or HTLV-III virus got into the homosexual community in America and from there spread around the world almost like a plague focussed in the drug culture and homosexual community. I think it was first its conventional venereal spread then probably spread from male prostitution to homosexuals extension by spread in the homosexual community coupled with spread from bisexuals to female sex partners or female drug addicts and then ultimately spread again to the heterosexual community which traces its current distribution. We now know from observations in Africa, Haiti, the United States and several other countries that this virus can be spread also from female to male and male to female in heterosexual prostitution. This presents the further problem of heterosexual transmission before us.

Wherever you talk to people these days they express deep concern about the many patients rapidly turning up with AIDS or ARC. Just how many of these persons there are and how many possible cases of AIDS will ultimately occur is guesswork. However, unless we can learn in some way how to cope with the virus itself or alternatively how to cope with the host immune response more effectively than we are now doing, at least 40-50,000 cases will occur even though we could immunize tomorrow. The number of patients will be large enough so that this epidemic will surely touch the lives of all of us.

I am finally convinced that Childhood AIDS described by Jim Olesky, Arye Rubinstein and Art Ammann and their co-workers earlier is a true entity. The presentation by S. Pahwa revealed clearly to me that this disease is not only a reality but also an awful one. Childhood AIDS now is a major cause of childhood immunodeficiency. Living in the relatively protected environment of the midwest, I wasn't seeing this extraordinary group of patients. Savita Pahwa's description, in this meeting, of the patients with Childhood AIDS who were well studied in virological as well as serological terms helped immensely in definition of the Childhood AIDS syndrome. One thing that really stood out in Dr. Pahwa's description is that children with AIDS do not ordinarily have agammaglobulinemia, hypogammaglobulinemia or even dysgammaglobulinemias as had been emphasized by others. Instead they have hypergammaglobulinemia. Hypergammaglobulinemia coupled with an antibody deficiency syndrome is the most common manifestation. Now that we have very specific diagnostic tools in the form of antibody responses to P_{41} and P_{24} antigens and virus isolation from peripheral blood lymphocytes to rely on the diagnosis of AIDS due to LAV or HTLV-III can be very certain. We no longer have to hazard lumping other immunodeficiency diseases with the AIDS and/or ARC children. AIDS in children is most serious and much worse than any have realized from earlier studies. Evidence of even horizontal transmission within families has been attributable by Pahwa to very close contact of children with parents. Perhaps exchange of saliva is responsible for this form of spread. So the challenge of AIDS, ARC and childhood AIDS grows and we still must stand quite helplessly by.

Will we ever be able to marshall an effective approach to cellular engineering to correct the immunodeficiency diseases of these unfortunate children such as was possible when we introduced bone marrow transplantation to cure SCID. Alternatively, all of the children who develop full blown AIDS must die of their immunodeficiency. Once the disease is expressed in its full bloom, treatment of the antibody deficiency component by administration of intravenous immunoglobulin preparations should be a good place to start in efforts to modify this relentless course. The IV immunoglobulin preparations are rapidly getting better and better and I think these preparations even now can be used in our AIDS patients to forestall opportunistic bacterial infections especially those attributable to the high grade encapsulated bacterial pathogens. Of course in these patients we must be alert for pneumocystis carinii pneumonia. This disease is very treatable when it occurs in children as a consequence of primary immunodeficiency diseases. Many SCID patients now have had pneumocystis treated first by trimethoprim sulfamethoxazole and later had their SCID corrected by marrow transplantation. If this order is followed, the SCID can be completely cured. However, if the pneumocystis carinii infection is not recognized or appreciated, correction of the immunodeficiency before the pneumocystis has been eliminated from the lungs may produce an overwhelming interstitial pneumonia--a veritable white-out that is rapidly lethal. This approach with trimethoprim sulfamethoxazole plus marrow transplantation is not attractive in AIDS because as the immunological correction would be made the persistant T_4 trophic virus will be expected to infect the newly developing T_4 cells. Recently, however, we have found in mice that we can introduce resistance genes against the mouse leukemia retrovirus or against retrovirus associated autoimmune diseases by bone marrow transplantation. Each of these diseases develop early in life, each leads to profound deficit of T-Lymphocytes and T-Lymphocyte function and each is associated with retrovirus infections. Yet by marrow transplantation we can correct every single abnormality in these animals. We accomplish this by transplanting the involved mice with marrow from inbred strains of mice that carry resistance genes. The transplants that are effective can be done either within or across major histocompatibility barriers. To achieve this feat requires tricks that we can't yet apply to man. For example, we may employ nude mice as the source of resistant cells using nude mice from strains with highly resistant backgrounds. Working in this context we have already repeatedly cured leukemia, autoimmune diseases and certain persistent virus infections in mice and the problems do not return. We can even correct all of the immunologic abnormalities that we see in the animals with these diseases. The abnormalities corrected include such abnormalities as early thymic involution and infiltration of thymus with B cells and plasma cells. We have even been able to cure the lymphoma-leukemia in mice when the thymus is already filled with leukemia or lymphomatous cells. Such susceptible mice, in whom resistance genes have been introduced by marrow transplantation, may have donor cells that are infected with the virus or viruses causative for the leukemia development after marrow transplantation or autoimmunity yet disease is not produced. These mice can have perfectly normal looking and normal functioning thymuses if we have given them appropriate bone marrow cells from donors resistant to the autoimmune or lymphomatous diseases in question. Thus, by marrow transplantation, we correct their thymus abnormalities their leukemias or autoimmunities and the abnormalities don't return. It has even been possible in experimental animals with autoimmune diseases or leukemia to wait until the disease has become well established, and still be able to correct the disease and all the immunologic abnormalities which feature propensity to develop disease in these mice. Thus, the essential components responsible for both autoimmune disease and leukemia appear to reside in radio-sensitive stem cells. If you introduce the appropriate radio-sensitive stem cells, bearing resistance genes, the viruses can't, by themselves, produce the destructive diseases. Thus, I believe that as we learn more about the natural history of AIDS, Childhood AIDS, and ARC, we will learn how to use cellular engineering perhaps by bone marrow transplantation from unrelated donors to introduce resistance genes against AIDS or ARC. It is already regularly possible to take marrow from resistant, mismatched donors made tolerant of recipient by repeated injection of recipient cells plus cyclophosphamide and then later, after purging the marrow of T-Lymphocytes, to do marrow transplants across major histocompatibility barriers without inducing GVHR. With such preparations we can reconstitute the entire hematopoietic systems, not have problems in the collaboration between the accessory cells and the B and T components of the specific immunity systems. With such preparations we can regularly introduce resistance genes across major histocompatibility barriers without producing GVHD. Similarly we can introduce resistance genes which permit treatment and cure of certain other virus-induced malignancies. We are now also testing the possibility of this approach to introduce resistance against chemical carcinogen-induced causes. From these experiments, although it will not be easy, we think it will not be impossible to identify and to introduce resistance genes by marrow transplantation in humans. Perhaps such resistance genes, if they can be identified, may inhibit persistence and progression of AIDS. This is a real challenge but I believe it will be impossible, now that the virus and its target cells are known.·

Dr. Greenspan and the Stanford group considered once again the pathogenesis of AIDS related refractory thrombocytopenia. He found that the thrombopenia in the AIDS patients he was considering to be attributable to auto-antibodies directed against the platelets rather than to circulating immunocomplexes which Karpatkin had earlier implicated in the pathogenesis of thrombopenia in AIDS. More work is needed but certainly the problem of thrombopenia represents a component of the AIDS Related Complex. How to approach this complication seems to be at issue. Here again my reaction is that we may not be using intravenous gammaglobulin nearly enough in patients with AIDS. Thrombopenic purpura in AIDS patients may be another indication for such treatment. IVIG provided surprisingly effective treatment for thrombopenias of chidren and adults that were first be treated by splenectomy and then by adrenal cortical steroids. Many such patients can now be treated with large doses of IVIG and nothing else. I don't think that we should be scared off by the few unexplained adverse reactions that have been described by the San Francisco group earlier. The patients with AIDS and ARC have antibody deficiency syndrome and we may be able to help those with thrombopenia especially by administration of the progressively improving intravenous gammaglobulin preparations that are now available. Dr. Pahwa's observations with Childhood AIDS are compatible with the view that intravenous gammaglobulin therapy can be useful also in preventing infections in patients with Childhood AIDS..

Yes, we, as scientists and scholars, have been treated well in this conference. We have learned many lessons and have much to take home to our laboratories and to our clinics. We have a great deal of work still to do. We have new drugs, new therapies, and new combinations of therapies to try. We can begin to think up strategies for treatment of ARC and perhaps even be able to prevent AIDS. We can visualize the development of better agents along lines already under consideration. Remember AIDS and ARC represent the greatest challenge facing clinical immunology today. Perhaps this epidemic represents the greatest challenge of immunology's entire 200 year history. Certainly it is the greatest immunologic challenge of my lifetime. I began my work in immunology in 1944, 40 years ago. Since then we have made astonishing progress. In 1944 we knew nothing of the cells, organs, molecules or genes involved in immunity. We have seen an extraordinary development of knowledge in but a few years. AIDS and ARC now threaten us, and these disorders caused by a retrovirus place the severest test of our understanding and ingenuity. What we are able to accomplish with the increasing understanding coming from improvements in our knowledge will only be told with time. The AIDS syndrome, its ARC and Childhood AIDS represent a real test of fire for modern immunology. The virus is at hand but we now must face the issue of heterosexual transmission, the threat of horizontal transmission as well as vertical transmission from mother to infant. Each represents a challenging problem and each will test our metal as immunologists, virologists, immunopharmacologists and cellular engineers. We must rise to the challenge. I feel certain we can and will. It was through the interfaces of virology and neurophysiology and I became an immunologist. As geneticists and immunologists we must develop skills that permit us to cope now with the virological threat before us. We need to be more than dualogists, we must be trilogists and more. I am sure that with an advancing pharmacology, immunopharmacology and cellular engineering we can lick the AIDS problem. The start is not bad and we have already had

as vertical transmission from mother to infant. Each represents a challenging problem and each will test our metal as immunologists, virologists, immunopharmacologists and cellular engineers. We must rise to the challenge. I feel certain we can and will. It was through the interfaces of virology and neurophysiology that I became an immunologist. As geneticists and immunologists we must develop skills that permit us to cope now with the virological threat before us. We need to be more than dualologists we must be trilogists and more. I am sure that with an advancing pharmacology, immunopharmacology and cellular engineering we can lick the AIDS problem. The start is not bad and we have already had glimpses of responses in our patients. Further with the virus at hand, AIDS no longer has to be mysterious or to seem unapproachable. We can learn how to prevent this disease. We will see soon antiviral vaccines that will prevent it. The virologists will give us that. But the cellular and humoral immunologists, immunopharmacologists and immunotherapists too must rise to the occasion so that we can learn to provide resistance that can halt the disease. With imaginative extension and development of our basic and applied sciences I believe we can learn to reconstruct the deficient immune system and/or introduce resistance genes so that we can save children and even adults who are otherwise doomed by their infection.

Once again we give our thanks to Dr. Sudhir Gupta, to each of the organizers, to all who supported and all who participated in this challenging conference. We especially need to thank one another for the criticisms and generated queries. The only true compliment scientists can give one another is to criticize the scientific efforts constructively. It is in this way that the work we do can be kept in best focus, the wit sharpened, and discoveries and understanding accelerated. Thanks again, Dr. Glasky, for your funding and continued enthusiasm. We need that too.

CONTRIBUTORS

Donald I. Abrams, San Francisco General Hospital, San Francisco, California.

Steven A. Armentrout, Division of Hematology/Oncology, University of California, Irvine, California.

Ellyn Ashida, UCLA Center for Health Sciences, Los Angeles, California.

Francoise Barre-Sinoussi, Unite'd'Oncologie Virale Institut Pasteur, Paris, France.

Gildon N. Beall, Harbor-UCLA Medical Center, Torrance, California.

J. George Bekesi, Department of Neoplastic Diseases, Mount Sinai School of Medicine, New York, New York.

E.L. Berrie, Departments of Immunology and Virology, St. Mary's Hospital Medical School, London, England.

Francoise Brun-Vezinet, Laboratoire de Virologic, Hospital Claude Bernard, Paris, France.

Dominic Casareale, Department of Pathology and Laboratory Medicine, University of Nebraska Medical Center, Omaha, Nebraska.

Jean-Claude Chermann, Unite'd'Oncologic Virale, Institut Pasteur, Paris, France.

Macus A. Conant, AIDS Clinical Research Center, University of California, San Francisco, California.

Susanna Cunningham-Rundles, Memorial Sloan-Kettering Cancer Center, New York, New York.

Kevin M. DeCock, USC Liver Unit, Rancho Los Amigos Hospital, Downey, California.

Lawrence Eppolito, UCLA Center for Health Sciences, Los Angeles, California.

John L. Fahey, UCLA Center for Health Sciences, Los Angeles, California.

Senih Fikrig, Department of Pediatrics, Downstate Medical Center, Brooklyn, New York.

Robert C. Gallo, Laboratory of Tumor Cell Biology, National Cancer Institute, National Institutes of Health, Bethesda, Maryland.

Robert A. Good, Department of Pediatrics, Oklahoma Medical Research Foundation, Oklahoma City, Oklahoma.

Michael S. Gottlieb, UCLA Center for Health Sciences, Los Angeles, California.

Deborah Greenspan, School of Dentistry and Medicine, University of California, San Francisco, California.

John S. Greenspan, School of Dentistry and Medicine, University of California, San Francisco, California.

Sudhir Gupta, Division of Basic and Clinical Immunology, University of California, Irvine, California.

Allan L. Goldstein, George Washington University Medical Center, Washington, D.C.

Beatrice Hahn, Laboratory of Tumor Cell Biology, National Cancer Institute, National Institutes of Health, Bethesda, Maryland.

J.R.W. Harris, Department of Immunology and Virology, St. Mary's Hospital Medical School, London, England.

David Hardy, UCLA Center for Health Sciences, Los Angeles, California.

G. Hayward, Memorial Sloan-Kettering Cancer Center, New York, New York.

D.J. Jeffries, Departments of Immunology and Virology, St. Mary's Hospital Medical School, London, England.

Ellen Kahn, North Shore University Hospital, Manhasset, New York.

Mark Kaplan, North Shore University Hospital, Manhasset, New York.

Craig M. Kessler, George Washington University Medical Center, Washington, D.C.

Dobri D. Kiprov, Children's Hospital of San Francisco, San Francisco, California.

Steven Knight, UCLA Center for Health Sciences, Los Angeles, California.

M. Krim, Memorial Sloan-Kettering Cancer Center, New York, New York.

Gerhard Krueger, Immunopathology Laboratories, Pathology Institute, University of Cologne, Cologne, West Germany.

Evelyne T. Lennette, Virolab, Emeryville, California.

Helen Lipscomb, Department of Pathology and Laboratory Medicine, University of Nebraska Medical Center, Omaha, Nebraska.

Phillip D. Markham, Laboratory of Tumor Cell Biology, National Cancer Institute, National Institutes of Health, Bethesda, Maryland.

Usha Mathur-Wagh, Department of Medicine, Beth Israel Medical Center, New York, New York.

C.E. Metroka, Memorial Sloan-Kettering Cancer Center, New York, New York.

Donna Mildvan, Department of Medicine, Beth Israel Medical Center, New York, New York.

Timothy Mess, San Francisco General Hospital, San Francisco, California.

Luc Montagnier, Unie'd'Oncologie Virale, Institut Pasteur, Paris, France.

Paul H. Naylor, George Washington University Medical Center, Washington, D.C.

Amit Patel, UCLA Center for Health Sciences, Los Angeles, California.

Rajendra Pahwa, North Shore University Hospital, Manhasset, New York.

Savita Pahwa, North Shore University Hospital, Manhasset, New York.

Anthony J. Pinching, Departments of Immunology and Virology, St. Mary's Hospital Medical School, London, England.

Vibeke H. Peterson, Virolab, Emeryville, California.

David T. Purtilo, Department of Pathology and Laboratory Medicine, University of Nebraska Medical Center, Omaha, Nebraska.

Julia P. Roboz, Department of Neoplastic Diseases, Mount Sinai School of Medicine, New York, New York.

Majorie Robert-Guroff, George Washington University Medical Center, Washington, D.C.

B.Y. Rubin, Memorial Sloan-Kettering Cancer Center, New York, New York.

L.A. Rogers, Departments of Immunology and Virology, St. Mary's Hospital Medical School, London, England.

S. Zaki-Salahuddin, Laboratory of Tumor cell Biology, National Cancer Institute, National Institutes of Health, Bethesda, Maryland.

M.G. Sarngadharan, Laboratory of Tumor Cell Biology, National Cancer Institute, National Institutes of Health, Bethesda, Maryland.

Bijan Safai, Memorial Sloan-Kettering Cancer Center, New York, New York.

Richard S. Schulof, George Washington University Medical Center, Washington, D.C.

George M. Shaw, Laboratory of Tumor Cell Biology, National Cancer Institute, National Institutes of Health, Bethesda, Maryland.

Gary L. Simon, George Washington University Medical Center, Washington, D.C.

Joseph Sonnabend, AIDS Medical Research Foundation, New York, New York.

Nora Sun, UCLA Center for Health Sciences, Los Angeles, California.

Ilya Spigland, Division of Virology, Montefiore Hospital and Medical Center, Bronx, New York.

Marcelo B. Sztein, George Washington University Medical Center, Washington, D.C.

Peter Tsang, Department of Neoplastic Diseases, Mount Sinai School of Medicine, New York, New York.

Paul A. Volberding, San Francisco General Hospital, San Francisco, California.

David J. Volsky, Department of Pathology and Laboratory Medicine, University of Nebraska Medical Center, Omaha, Nebraska.

J.N. Weber, Departments of Immunology and Virology, St. Mary's Hospital Medical School, London, England.

Constance Wofsy, AIDS Clinical Research Center, University of California, San Francisco, California.

Peter R. Wolfe, UCLA Center for Health Sciences, Los Angeles, California.

INDEX

MIX
Papier aus verantwortungsvollen Quellen
Paper from responsible sources
FSC® C105338

If you have any concerns about our products,
you can contact us on
ProductSafety@springernature.com

In case Publisher is established outside the EU,
the EU authorized representative is:
Springer Nature Customer Service Center GmbH
Europaplatz 3, 69115 Heidelberg, Germany

Printed by Libri Plureos GmbH
in Hamburg, Germany